Why Am I So Miserable If These Are the Best Years of My Life?

Why Am I So Miserable If These Are the Best Years of My Life?

A SURVIVAL GUIDE FOR THE YOUNG WOMAN

BY *Andrea Boroff Eagan*

WITH AN INTRODUCTION BY *Ellen Frankfort*

J. B. LIPPINCOTT COMPANY   *Philadelphia and New York*

The illustrations on pages 122, 124, 132, 134, 140, 148, 151, 155, and 168 are by Russell Hoover.

U.S. Library of Congress Cataloging in Publication Data

Eagan, Andrea Boroff, birth date
Why am I so miserable if these are the best years of my life?

Bibliography: p.
Includes index.
SUMMARY: A guide to help the teenage girl learn who she is and what she wants, avoid a few pitfalls, and learn the facts she needs to make decisions.
1. Sex instruction for girls. 2. Adolescent girls—Juvenile literature. 3. Etiquette for children and youth. [1. Sex instruction for girls. 2. Adolescence] I. Title.
HQ35.E17   301.43'15   75-43726
ISBN-0-397-31655-0

This book is for my mother,
Dorothy Protter Boroff,
and my father,
Daniel A. Boroff.

Acknowledgments

To Ellin Hirst, Lynn Phillips, and Marcia Salo Rizzi, who helped me to understand what it means to be a woman.

To Susan Ann Protter, my agent, who said, "Of course you can."

To Ann Kearns, who was willing to gamble.

To Dorothy Briley and Ellen Stuttle of J. B. Lippincott Company, for their enthusiasm, editorial guidance, and good work.

To Barbara Clum and Jeanne A. Glass of Pyramid Publications, for their help and concern.

To my gynecologist, Dr. Marcia L. Storch, for always answering my questions and for being an example of just how good a doctor can be. Any errors that remain in the medical material (or anywhere else) are my responsibility and are there because I didn't have the sense to ask.

To Rena Uviller of the American Civil Liberties Union, for reviewing the legal material. Again, any errors are my own.

To the women of the Women's Health Organizing Collective and HealthRight, especially Pamela Booth, Naomi Fatt, and Rachel Fruchter, for never-failing support.

To Madeline Belkin, for reading portions of the manuscript and for making a number of excellent suggestions.

To all the women and men who helped to take care of Molly, making it possible for me to write, especially Carol Brightman and Richard Levy.

To all the women I've taught and counseled in the past few years, from whom I learned much more than they did from me.

To Richard, who put me and this book back together more than once, for love, encouragement, and caring, and for believing in me.

Contents

Introduction

Cream-colored convertibles. I'll never forget them. No, I didn't lose "it" (my virginity) in one; but I spent an entire summer when I was a teenager counting cream-colored convertibles. I can still remember the excitement when I hit one hundred, about late July. But as I got into the one hundred forties, it was no longer excitement that I felt; it was more like I was going crazy. I was almost there—at the magical number that would determine the rest of my life. All I had to do was reach one hundred and fifty, and then the next boy who spoke to me would be The One I would marry and settle down with for the rest of my life. And, of course, we'd live happily forever after.

It's curious that now I can't even remember who the boy turned out to be, although I can vividly recall sitting on the stoop and screaming out "Here comes another!" and adding one more cream-colored convertible to the careful count we kept. (I wasn't the only one doing this; all the girls in my neighborhood were similarly occupied.) What an ingenious scheme to keep teenage girls busy. Even the timing was perfect. In the early 1950s it took just about an entire summer to count one hundred and fifty cream-colored convertibles, if you devoted every day to it and kept on the lookout even when you were not officially sitting and keeping count.

Only now, when I look back, can I see the grotesqueness of it all: thousands of teenage girls sitting and counting cars—never questioning why, taking it all so seriously—never once thinking there might be a better way to spend our time, even though not one of us really believed that the first boy who spoke to us at the end of the count would be The One. Grotesque as it was, it used up time and energy while we got our first taste of fantasy built around romance.

Unfortunately, a lot of those girls grew up continuing to think about romance with all the energy and passion with which they once counted cars. Many of them are now the mothers of teenage daughters, but they have never grown out of their obsession with romance, and obsessions seldom have much to do with reality. They dream about the delivery boy or the cute young doctor on a daytime serial—rarely about their husbands. Others managed to put away their adolescent obsession with romance by repressing their feelings. The women who grew up to have healthy adult relationships will almost always tell you that growing up was very, very painful.

All this is why I got so excited while reading *Why Am I So Miserable If These Are the Best Years of My Life?* If only I could have read, when I was first falling in love, "Love doesn't have to last forever in order to be 'real love.' " Andrea Eagan offers a well-balanced, realistic view of the world in this book. Her advice is wise and understanding—yet she is never preachy. She points out that with a first love, "you probably feel sure that it's going to last forever. You might (though the chances are slim) continue to love your first love for the rest of your life." Andrea never insists that something is impossible; she just points out what is likely to happen.

"You also can't prove to someone that you love him by doing something for him." Now there's a line I wish all my girlfriends and I had had to memorize. Everything we had learned told us just the opposite: Please a man, wait for *him* to call or you may scare him; and whatever you do, don't appear smarter than he is, men don't like that. In other words, we were never to show our real selves. No wonder men didn't think of us as real!

This book is written, as you will see, from the vantage point of now. Andrea knows all the lines boys have used in the past to get girls to do what they didn't want to do but felt pressured into doing for "his" sake. In fact, there was nostalgia for me in remembering all the silly rituals and taboos. On the first date, you kissed; on the second, you necked; on the third, you started to pet above the waist. Although sex was based on rules and treated as a game, it was a very serious one. To say "sex doesn't necessarily have to do with love" was unthinkable. Only now does it seem reasonable to admit what, in fact, has always been true. It's possible to love someone and not want to have sex; to have unsatisfying sex and still love someone; to have great sex with someone you're not in love with. All of these were unthinkable combinations only a decade or two ago.

And about sex itself—I remember Miss Barrett, my sixth-grade teacher, calling me to her desk and whispering that I was to take a book to the rest room and erase a passage that had been scribbled in red pencil at the top of a page. The passage read: *Stick your penis in her vagina and wind up with a brat.* I was as horrified as Miss Barrett that someone would write such a thing in a reader, but (and this is even more horrifying) it was the clearest description of the sex act I had received. I had been given loads of books about birds and bees and frogs and fish, but I had never been told exactly what went where. I figured the water took care of everything with the fish, and all the rest was a mystery. You can imagine how I reacted when I read the clear, precise descriptions of the sex act in this book.

The one area that Andrea discusses here that is *not* nostalgic to recall is women at work. The subject was hardly ever mentioned when I was growing up. We were all going to get married, even if it wasn't to the first boy who came along after we'd finished counting convertibles. The truth is—and Andrea points it out very well—that women have always worked; we just haven't always gotten credit for it. The times we live in are filled with change. I suspect that fewer and fewer girls will automatically respond to the what-are-you-going-to-be question with "Housewife and mother" (any more than boys would answer, "Househusband and father"). And as the thought of spending an entire summer counting one hundred and fifty cream-colored convertibles becomes more ludicrous, fewer girls will be wondering, "If these are the best years of my life, why am I so miserable?"

Ellen Frankfort

Why Am I So Miserable If These Are the Best Years of My Life?

1

Just Be Yourself

Someone, at some time, has probably told you to "just be yourself." That's a timeworn cliché that sounds perfectly simple, even logical. Obviously, everyone should know how to be herself. But it's not that easy. If it were easy, you would never have to wonder how to act in a new situation, and you'd never feel confused about your feelings. But being yourself isn't any more automatic than playing tennis or driving a car or reading. First you have to learn the basics and then you have to practice. You also have to be aware of whatever you're doing, so that you can recognize your mistakes and correct them. You shouldn't expect to know exactly what to do the first time you're exposed to a new situation. And if you're nervous, it's going to be even harder to sort out your feelings and figure out how you want to act. While you're a teenager, you'll be having new experiences and new feelings all the time. You won't be able to handle everything perfectly the first time

—or at any time—and you shouldn't expect to. But you can use these years to learn a lot about yourself.

Getting to know who you are and how to be yourself is a lifelong process. It began soon after you were born, when you first learned that there was a difference between your body and the world outside your skin. If you work at it, you'll continue to learn things about yourself no matter how long you live. No one ever completely figures herself out. There are always surprises left. So if tomorrow someone tells you to "be yourself" and you don't know how and you're not sure what that means, don't worry about it. There's no easy way to find out who you are.

Once in a while, you'll read a magazine article with a title like "What Type Are You?" and a list of twenty questions or so, asking things like, "Do you enjoy taking long walks, or would you rather read?" But you are much more complicated than the answers to those questions. And besides, you are constantly changing, while the choice of answers always seems to stay the same.

No one knows more about you than you know yourself, even though some people may try to tell you that they do. A friend may say, "You always know what to say to boys," or, "You can't keep a secret." Or your mother may say, "You're too young to understand," or, "You never think for yourself" (even if she always tries to do your thinking for you). Other people can and will make judgments about and for you. What others have to say may be valuable—or it may be absolutely wrong. While it's helpful to know what others think of you, in the end you're the one who has to decide what's right and what's wrong for you. You know when you're enjoying yourself; when you're uncomfortable; when you're acting phony; when you don't understand something. In fact, you probably already know a lot more about yourself than you think you do.

How others see us is always interesting and is sometimes useful in helping us to see ourselves clearly. Every time someone tells you something— "You're never on time," or, "You're not good enough to be on the basketball team"—stop and decide whether they're right or wrong. You can look for patterns, too. The things your friends tell you may be an indication of certain behavior patterns you've been trying to discard or don't truly understand. But don't measure things you do through your friends' eyes. Remember they may see what you do, but you're the only one who knows or can find out why you do them.

When you honestly don't know what you feel or think about something, it's important to admit, at least to yourself, that you are confused. When you really don't know what to do or think, it's reasonable to accept the judgment of someone you respect, provided her or his advice makes sense for you. Accepting someone else's judgment and going along with the crowd, however, are two totally different things.

Accepting someone's judgment requires careful thinking about the issue, whatever it is. Going along with the crowd usually means that you're not thinking at all about what you're doing.

One thing you can do to get to know yourself better is to experiment with different *roles.* You can try out being mysterious and sophisticated; or quiet and intellectual; or bouncy and enthusiastic; or just plain tough. Or anything else you can think of. Some of the things you try will feel comfortable and will stick. Others will require too much effort or will make you feel uncomfortable. Adopting and keeping up a personality that is completely out of tune with who you usually are (that is, one that is neither comfortable nor natural) is impossible for most people. But trying out different roles—different ways of acting and speaking—is perfectly natural. You can keep what you like, what feels right for you, and discard what you don't like. Eventually you'll find that there are all sorts of ways of being who you are. You don't have to be any one way all the time, and you don't have to try to live up to what anyone else thinks you should be.

Making Changes

You've probably already found out that you can't change someone who doesn't want to be changed. You can change yourself if you want to, even though it's not always easy. Change and growth will continue to happen to you for the rest of your life. If you really want to, you can have control over the kind and direction of change that you go through, so that (just possibly) you can become older and wiser, instead of only older.

Whether you are open with other people or reserved, timid or aggressive, short-tempered or calm, outgoing or solitary, cautious or trusting—these characteristics are basic to you by now. But if there are things about yourself that you don't like, you can usually do something about them, no matter how basic they may seem. You have to be able, first of all, to recognize your strengths and your weaknesses. Do you make friends easily, for example, or does it take a long time for you to overcome your shyness? Are you likely to express your opinion about something, or do you tend to keep your mouth shut and let other people think you agree with them? Once you've become aware of how you usually act, then and only then can you start to make decisions about what you're content with and what you'd like to change. Be realistic. Don't waste your time wishing that your eyes were a different color, or that you were a foot taller, or that your father was rich. There's nothing you can do about those things. But if you wish you had lots of friends, then you can at least muster your courage and go out and make one friend.

Though it may sound contradictory, you have to like yourself and accept yourself before you can make successful changes. Liking yourself doesn't mean you have to think you're perfect or that there's nothing about yourself you wish were different. For instance, suppose you know someone who is painfully shy and uncomfortable in groups. She's relaxed and friendly with one or two people, but as soon as she gets into a crowd she fades into the wall. If you don't like her because she can't get along in a crowd and you put her down for that, it isn't going to help her much. In fact, it's only going to make her feel more of a failure and act more insecure in a situation which is already difficult for her. But if you like her as she is and accept her as a human being, then you may be able to help her. Once she knows that she's liked and understood as she is, she has an incentive to develop and change.

Now, try to apply the same reasoning to yourself. If you don't like yourself and are always putting yourself down, it's going to be hard for you to believe that you can make any changes or improvements. If you can accept that you're really okay as you are, but you'd like to be a better "you," you have a chance. After all, there's at least as much good about you as there is about anyone else.

Making Decisions

Part of learning to be yourself involves learning to make decisions for yourself. There are times when it's hard to know exactly what you want to do or what would be best for you, especially when major decisions have to be made. But if you start making decisions about little things, you'll get the experience you need to help you make bigger decisions. Any decision, no matter how trivial it seems, is important. If you decide to buy a pair of shoes because you like the way they look though you suspect they might turn out to be uncomfortable, and if they *are* uncomfortable, then you've learned something. If you eat too much or drink too much, and you get sick, you've learned something too. That doesn't necessarily mean that you won't make the same mistake again. No one is quite so smart that she never makes the same mistake twice. Or three times. Or even more. What you do eventually learn is that every decision has consequences and that you have to take the possible consequences into account before you make the decision.

Part of making a decision involves recognizing the number of choices that are really available. There are usually more possibilities in a situation than you can see at first glance. If it's time to register for classes at school and you have to choose one elective course and can't make up your mind between typing and Spanish, stop and think about it for a while. It may be that you really need to know how to type and that you can get along without knowing Spanish (or the other way around). Or there may be some other course that you prefer altogether. But try to make the decision on your own. Don't take typing just because your best friend is taking it; don't take Spanish because some boy you're interested in might be in your class. If you take any subject for any reason other than because you're interested in learning about it, you make a mistake, and most of all you do yourself out of what might be an interesting experience.

There are relatively few decisions that can't be changed. Once you realize that you've made a mistake, more often than not you can change what you're doing, if you stop to think about it. Naturally, the sooner you recognize your mistake, the easier it will be to shift gears. Just because you've started something, doesn't automatically mean that you have to go through with it. It is, of course, a good habit to finish what you start. However, if in your second year of high school you decide you should be taking an academic course instead of a commercial course, there's probably a way to change your program, if you're determined enough.

Making decisions and learning from them, both the successes and the mistakes, develops your judgment. Judgment is simply the ability to make good decisions. As your judgment develops until you can make decisions you're reasonably sure are right for you, you'll gradually learn to trust your decision-making ability.

An important part of knowing yourself lies in knowing how to make the right decisions for yourself. And being yourself means, at least in part, being willing to act on the decisions that you know are right.

Being Different

One of the things that you'll find affects your decisions is pressure from your social group. It's always tempting, because it's usually easiest, to conform to whatever your particular crowd is doing or thinking. And doing something that goes against the crowd means taking the risk of being considered different, which is a difficult thing to do. If your friends are going to cut you out because you don't always go along with them, you're going to find yourself, sooner or later, facing some very tough choices. You're going to have to make your choices based on your judgments of what is right for you, not for your friends. The only thing that can make those choices a little easier is your determination to do whatever is best for you, even if it is unpopular.

It's unlikely, of course, that your friends are going to drop you because of your opinions about minor things, like whether or not you like pizza or whether or not *Billy Jack* is your all-time favorite movie. So you can get some practice at expressing your opinions on things like that without taking any great risk. And that may make it a little easier to be honest about a difference of opinion on the bigger things. It's also entirely possible that once you've broken the ice, other people will feel freer about expressing

their real opinions—and then you can all stop believing that everyone thinks the same about everything.

It's doubtful that you always want to be exactly
like everyone else. And you shouldn't expect anyone
else to be exactly like you either. You have to learn to
give your friends room to be different and not put
them down for it. Respecting other people's actions
and feelings and opinions when they differ from
your own doesn't mean that you don't have strong
values of your own.

Respecting other people doesn't mean either that
you can't try to change someone else's mind about
something. But first you have to try to understand
why she says or thinks the things she does. You need
to be flexible and honest enough to change when
you realize that you are wrong, or you can't expect
the same from anyone else. And you must have
enough courage and care enough about someone
else to try to persuade her to change if the matter is
really important. You're not going to waste your time
trying to get your friend to like a pair of shoes that
she hates. Her taste in clothes or food or movies
shouldn't matter to you, if you have more important
things in common. But if you think she's making
herself unhappy by allowing her boyfriend to put
her down in public, you might want to try talking to
her.

You Are What You Choose

Knowing who you are can be complicated by the

fact that you act differently in different situations. When you go to visit your grandmother, you probably talk, sit, dress, and eat differently than you do when you're hanging out with your best girlfriend. There's nothing dishonest about that. Nearly everyone acts differently in different situations. Being yourself does not mean being the same all the time.

Different people will expect different things of you, and it's never going to be possible for you to meet everyone's expectations all the time. Your girlfriend may assume that you'll always lend her your homework; your boyfriend may expect that you'll always agree to whatever he decides to do; and your parents may think that you're going to get a job after high school instead of going to college. There are times when it is going to seem easier to go along with whatever someone else wants or expects from you than to put up a fight for whatever you want. The danger is that if you always go along with what others want, you eventually get so out of touch with what *you* want and how *you* feel that you lose track of yourself. This doesn't mean that you should never do something for someone else's sake or that you can't ever compromise, but if you are compromising, you should at least know that you're doing it.

The major decisions of your life, however, should not be the place for compromise. If you really want to go to college, in spite of your family's objections, that's the time to fight for what you want. Or if everyone you know, including your boyfriend, assumes that you're going to get married right after graduation (because you've been going steady for six years), and if you have a sneaking suspicion that marriage might not be such a terrific idea right now, then you'd better follow your instincts. Even if it will be difficult to explain to everyone.

Choosing Your Friends

You probably don't like everyone you meet. If you're like most people, you immediately like some people, instantly dislike others, and don't feel much one way or the other about the rest. If you don't like everyone, then why do you want everyone to like you? Everyone is not going to want to be your friend, no matter what you do. If you go around being totally agreeable to everyone just so they'll like you, you're bound to run into at least one person who can't stand you because you don't seem to have a mind of your own.

What you can count on is that most people will have the same reaction to you that you have to them. Therefore, if you immediately take to someone when you meet her, the chances are good that she feels the same about you. That doesn't always work, of course, but you'd have to be ridiculously unlucky to find that you only liked people who didn't like you. Since most people want to be liked and want to have friends, we all tend to like the people who like us.

If you meet someone who seems to dislike you

right from the start, you may want to have her for a friend because you feel that she'd really be a friend worth having. But if you try to make a friend of her just because of the challenge, or because you can't stand having someone dislike you, then you're wasting your time. You're being dishonest. And if the feeling of dislike is mutual, then you really shouldn't care about it anyway.

Trying to make everyone else like you, or trying to do what everyone else wants you to do, or trying to act like someone you're not is eventually self-defeating. It takes up all your energy and meanwhile does nothing for your self-respect or for your growth as a person. Your main job is to get in touch and stay in touch with your own feelings, and with your strengths, weaknesses, and abilities. That's what it means to "just be yourself."

2

Who Do They Want You to Be?

You've probably already noticed that someone or other is nearly always telling you how to act or what to say or what to think or what you're supposed to be. Most of the time that doesn't help you figure out who you really are. Your parents tell you how nice (they think) teenagers acted when your parents were young. Your boyfriend tells you what to do. Television, radio, magazines, books, and newspapers, especially in their advertising, tell you how you should look and act. And they're all telling you something different. Your mother is telling you that nice girls don't do "those things"; and your boyfriend is telling you that everybody does it. Revlon is pushing the "natural look," while Coty just came out with a new line of black-and-blue lipstick

If everyone were telling you the same thing, it would be easier to cope. You'd only have to decide whether or not to go along. But with everyone telling you different things, it's often difficult to sort out which advice you want to take and which you don't. It doesn't get you anywhere to resist one set of demands and then unconsciously go along with another. If you decide that you don't care to wear whatever's the latest thing, that doesn't mean you have to insist on wearing jeans to your sister's wedding.

One of the first things you can do when you find yourself faced with conflicting pressures is try to figure out why a particular pressure is being put on you. Then you can decide for yourself whether or not you want to go along with it, though that's seldom as simple as it sounds. When you're a teenager, it's sometimes impossible to do what *you* think you should or what you've decided would be best for you. And it's hard to learn to think for yourself when everyone around is telling you what to think. A fashion magazine might tell you that this month you simply can't get along without purple eye shadow and green mascara. Your mother freaks out at the idea. Your girlfriend is wearing it. What do you do? First, you have to keep in mind that the company that sells the stuff doesn't care how *you* look. They're in business to make money, and by next month they'll be trying to sell you something else. Your mother may object to extreme makeup on you because it reminds her of the fact that you're growing up, which makes her feel old. Or maybe she thinks you're prettier without it. She may also not like to see you wasting money. And maybe your girlfriend always has to be the first to try anything new, no matter how it looks. None of those things should determine what you do about green mascara (or anything else). You have to decide what looks good on you, what you can afford, whether it's worth fighting with your mother about, and what you feel comfortable with. Then, if you really want to, you can go ahead and paint your whole face green.

Who Made You What You Are Today?

The first (and for a long time, the only) influence on a baby is the family into which she's born. Your family remains important in shaping how you think and act, and how you look at the world, even as you get older and become more independent. For instance, if your mother is always very neat and clean and insists that you be that way too, you'll probably find that you'll go back and forth between being very neat and very messy (as a rebellion against her) for many years until you reach the particular balance that works best for you.

If you have a brother, you've probably noticed that you and he are treated differently by your family. If your family is like most, he's probably not expected to help out in the kitchen, for example, but you are. And he probably has more privileges than you do, because your parents are not as strict with him. The different ways that boys and girls are raised start when they are tiny infants. If you look for it, you'll see that people treat boy babies and girl babies very differently. Girls are handled more gently and talked to more softly than boys, even when they're only a month old.

It may eventually be found that there are inborn differences between males and females that make us act in certain ways, but no one has proved that yet. More important than any inborn difference is the training you get. Little girls are often dressed in pretty dresses and expected to keep themselves clean, while little boys are expected to get filthy. A little girl gets what she wants by being cute and coy and flirty, while a boy's parents will encourage him to stand up for himself and simply ask for what he wants. If someone hits a little girl, it's accepted if she cries and runs to someone for comforting; but if someone hits a little boy, he's told, "Big boys don't cry," and, "Well, hit him back!" Girls learn early that being rough and aggressive isn't considered "right."

The toys that we're given to play with also reinforce all the other training that we get. Girls are given dolls and toy kitchens. Boys get trucks and helicopters. And you can often see a parent in a toy department saying to a little girl, "No, you can't have a truck. Trucks are for boys." Or saying to a boy, "No, you can't have a doll. Dolls are for girls." We quickly learn what we're going to be allowed to be interested in, and many of us never get the chance to explore the rest of the world.

Because unfeminine or "tomboy" behavior is discouraged, many girls lose the chance to discover and develop those parts of their personalities that are not thought to be typically "feminine." And the reverse is true for boys. A boy who is stopped from cuddling the doll he wants may never get the chance to express his feelings of tenderness and gentleness, since they're not considered "masculine." There is nothing *wrong* with the traits that are thought to be "feminine" or "masculine." What is wrong is that what we're allowed to be is limited by the standards of masculinity and femininity.

Learning to Be Female

When children start school, the ways that they're allowed to act remain different for boys and girls. Girls are expected to behave better, which usually means that girls are more likely to do what the teacher wants, while boys are more likely to "act up." Girls also learn more quickly than boys in the early grades and, on the whole, do better than boys at everything except sports. And we play sports poorly only because we're usually not encouraged to play well.

Girls and boys are taught to read from the same books. But even the books that we learn to read from emphasize and reinforce the standard male and female roles. The boys in the books do things; the girls watch the boys: "Look, Jane. See Dick jump." Women in early readers appear only as mothers; boys are shown helping their fathers. In fact, what men and women, or boys and girls, do is much more narrow and limited in these books than it is in most families.

By the age of six or so, most little girls are used to the idea that girls can do some things and boys can do others. Then two important things happen to girls, usually around the seventh grade. One is that we start being tracked into "girls'" subjects, like home economics and typing. The other is that we start to do worse than boys in school subjects.

There's nothing wrong with learning the things that you learn in home economics. Everyone, male and female, should know how to sew on a button and put together a decent meal. But it's just as necessary for everyone to know how to hang a shelf and fix a light switch. Unfortunately, in almost every school, only the girls learn about cooking and sewing, and only the boys learn about carpentry and electricity.

In many schools, even today, a girl isn't *allowed* to take shop courses. And if she wants vocational training of some kind, the only courses she can take are commercial courses. A girl in an academic program is often talked out of taking physics or Russian, and winds up taking French and biology instead, because physics and Russian are considered less "feminine" than French and biology. Girls in a lot of places have started to rebel against this kind of tracking and have often been successful, but it usually takes time and determination to win.

Since no one has found any connection between the onset of menstruation and the beginning of mental deterioration, there must be some other reason why girls' grades start to slip around the time they start junior high. One reason is that if a girl doesn't think she's going to have a career, it will hardly seem worth it to her to work hard learning things she'll never use. So if you're like most girls and expect to get married and not have to work outside your home, or to work for only a short time, you may very well not see the point of studying history or biology. The other thing that is likely to happen around the time you start junior high is that you start getting interested in boys—and you learn very fast that most boys don't like girls who are "brains." So if you feel that it's really important that you have a boyfriend, you're not going to want to look too smart.

What Is a Woman?

The ideal American girl is supposed to be popular, which means that she's supposed to have a date with an attractive boy every night, or every weekend at least. A popular girl has lots of friends, has the right clothes for every occasion, and never worries about doing the right thing. Besides that, she never gets depressed, never loses her temper, and never does anything that she's going to regret later.

Of course, the *ideal* American girl doesn't exist except in the imagination of novelists and magazine editors. No one is completely free of problems or pimples. No one is that self-assured, either, especially not as a teenager. It isn't even clear that the ideal teenager *should* exist, since no one is completely sure there are any benefits in being that popular. Even the girls (and boys) who are considered Most Popular worry about themselves, and about how they look and how they're supposed to act, and are constantly afraid of losing their cool and of losing their popularity. The girls who are popular as teenagers aren't any happier or more successful as they get older than those girls who have social problems in their teen years.

The pressure to be popular puts you in the bind of trying to have everyone like you. The fact that you are or are not "popular" (whatever you think that means and however important you think it is) doesn't really say much about who you are. It's more important for you to have a few good friends with whom you're comfortable than it is for you to have a whole lot of shallow relationships. It's terribly important that you not try to judge yourself by some impossible standard of popularity or beauty or other superficial gauge. Having lots of dates may be fine, but if you're bored or uncomfortable, or if you feel like you're wasting your time, then there's not much point to having the dates to begin with. Your free time is limited, and you have to decide how it's most important for you to spend it. Winning popularity contests doesn't mean anything in the long run; being envied by other people doesn't mean that you have friends; and being asked out every night doesn't mean that you're loved.

The Perfect Woman

If you look at the ads in the magazines, you probably get the idea that the advertisers are trying to tell you that the way to get love and be popular is to use their products. A lot of the advertising that's directed at women is designed to make us anxious about the way we look. And the more anxious we feel, the more likely we are to think we need things that promise to make us beautiful. It's a full-time job to keep yourself looking like a fashion model, and very expensive besides. It's actually less work in the long run to learn to accept yourself as you are and like it. That doesn't mean that you won't dress to look nice or that you'll never use makeup. But clothes and makeup should be thought of as decoration, not as necessary parts of your personality (which is not to say that you can get away with going around naked because that's what expresses you best). A lot of girls (and older women) simply won't go out of the house without makeup. You can't possibly look so different without your makeup, though, that you need to be so dependent on it. Advertising, of course, encourages you to be dependent on products—cosmetics, clothes, deodorants, perfumes, mouthwashes, hair sprays, etc., etc., etc.

Women today are expected to have hairless (except on our heads, of course), odorless, pimple-free, very soft, fatless bodies. All this is a matter of fashion and will probably change sooner or later, if that's any consolation. The test of what you do to yourself with cosmetics is a question of what *you* feel is necessary. A lot of women, for instance, don't mind hair on their legs, finding it less obnoxious than razor cuts, stubble, or smelly depilatories. If you find your own smell offensive, or if you perspire so much that you ruin your clothes, then a deodorant or antiperspirant is useful. However, for some people washing is sufficient, and certainly cheaper.

Some products are simply silly and expensive. Others, however, are downright dangerous. Some brands of makeup contain traces of metals, such as copper, zinc, lead, and mercury, which can be absorbed through the skin and can be harmful to your health. Another example is vaginal (or "feminine") deodorant. This is a new invention, and until some drug company thought it up, it never occurred to most women that they needed such a thing. In fact, a smelly discharge from the vagina that doesn't clear up when you wash with soap and water is a sign of infection and should send you to a doctor, not to a "feminine hygiene deodorant." In addition to covering up a condition that calls for medical treatment, vaginal deodorants can cause irritation and allergic reactions. They dry up your natural secretions, and some of them are made with talc,which may contain asbestos. Since asbestos seems to be linked to certain kinds of cancer, you're really better off not taking chances by spraying your crotch, or anywhere else for that matter, with a product containing talcum powder. (Some talcum powders do not contain asbestos, but unless you're sure a particular brand does not, it's best not to take a chance.) If you perspire so much that it makes you uncomfortable, a light dusting of plain cornstarch will help keep you dry.

The big push today is toward the "natural look." In *Seventeen* magazine, you can usually find a picture of a model with the natural look. Under the picture is a long paragraph describing how to use eight or ten different products to get the same natural look for yourself. It always seems to involve eye shadow, eyeliner, highlighter, mascara, base, blusher, lipstick, and lip gloss in two different shades. When you realize that all this means an investment of at least twenty dollars (just for your *face*), you begin to see the point. And next month, they're pushing new products and new colors, so you have to spend even more. The natural look can't mean simply having clean skin, clean hair, and no makeup, because if it did, the cosmetics manufacturers would all go broke. So they have to turn the natural look into a complicated ritual to get you to buy their products.

Recently, the word "natural" has been used to promote just about everything that's advertised on television: foods, makeup, hair dye, girdles, and fur-

niture polish. The advertisers seem to want us to get
the idea that if we use the natural products they're
selling, we'll wind up looking like the model in the
commercial. And in most of the "natural product"
commercials, the model is extremely thin and very
long-legged, and she tosses her head around so
much that it's a wonder she hasn't had to be hospi-
talized with a neck injury. You can eat Dannon yo-
gurt, use Natural Wonder makeup, and dye your hair
with Clairol, and you're still not going to come out
looking like that model—unless you looked that way
to start with, which most of us don't. But after the
message has been repeated time and time again, it's
hard not to get the idea that if you just use the right
product, you'll wind up being better off than you
already are.

Advertising encourages us to be dissatisfied with
the way we look and plays on our desire to be attractive. Beyond that, it is often insulting to our intelli-
gence. Women are supposed to be so unable to think
for themselves that, in the ads for floor cleaners and
detergents, for example, there's usually a man's
voice in the background telling the woman she's
right to be using that particular product. For about
ten years now, Josephine the Plumber, instead of
fixing anyone's plumbing, has been scrubbing sinks
and helping an occasional harried husband to wash
the piled-up dishes. Imagine a TV commercial in
which someone asked a male plumber to scour the
sink!

Women are shown in TV commercials getting other people to eat, worrying about "ring around the collar" and dirty floors, and taking care of other people's illnesses. If women are shown working, they're almost always secretaries and waitresses. Many women are good secretaries and good waitresses. Many women are good homemakers and good mothers. But many women are also good reporters or good doctors, and happy with what they do, and you almost never see them in commercials. And, not all women are married. In fact, a good many women are happy not being married, but you don't see them represented in TV commercials either. The point is not that TV shouldn't show women being housewives or secretaries, since in fact many women are housewives or secretaries. But it's got to be hard for you to want to be a lawyer unless you see that women can be lawyers and that a lot of lawyers are women.

Women's magazines don't do much better than television. Most magazines oriented specifically toward women are devoted either to fashion or to homemaking, but it's not unusual anymore for a women's magazine to carry a profile of a successful woman or a "serious" article about politics or health. All the same, most of their space is still devoted to advertising cosmetics or clothes or detergents. Quite often women are written about in these magazines because of the men that they're attached to, instead of because of who they are. There'll be an

interview with some politician's or golfer's wife or
with some ex-president's daughter, but the interview
is not about who that woman is or what she thinks.
She talks about her husband (or father) and what he
does, about her special recipe (*his* favorite), or about
how she keeps her hair neat when she has such a
busy schedule following him around. The fact that
any of these women may be interesting on their own
or may think things that aren't exactly the same as
what their men think is rarely taken into account.

A few pages of a magazine or one TV commercial
or an occasional TV situation comedy that puts wom-
en down could be ignored. What can't be ignored,
when it's constant, is the message, repeated again
and again and again, that women are not very interesting, not very bright, only good as props for
clothes and makeup, only interested in their appearance and their houses. The effect, in the end, can be
devastating for a woman's self-image. It's very hard
for any woman to hear this all the time and keep
from believing it eventually.

There have been films that showed women as
competent, independent human beings. In *Adam's
Rib,* made in the 1940s, for instance, Katharine Hepburn plays a defense attorney; her husband is a pros-
ecutor. Since they're involved in the same case, the
competition between them is open and fierce, both
in the courtroom and at home. And Hepburn is never made to appear either stupid or "unfeminine." In
too many movies, however, the image of women is

not very flattering. In fact, in many movies today, there are no women at all in important roles. The women are victims, prostitutes, and dingbats.

In films men are often shown as heroes, as people who control their own lives. Women are rarely shown that way in movies today. The men in films act out fantasies about masculinity. Everyone knows that Shaft and James Bond aren't realistic. Everyone understands that in real life the cop doesn't always solve the case, the doctor doesn't always cure the patient, and the pilot doesn't always land the plane safely. The way men are depicted isn't realistic. But the fantasy is a positive one: men are made to look better than they are. Women, though, are repeatedly made to look worse than they actually are. If the men are made larger than life, then the women are made smaller. Once again, a young girl has no image to fantasize herself into. It's hard to imagine yourself being a heroine if you've never seen anyone be one.

Feminine/Masculine

Today, the definition of what is "feminine" is changing. But the old definition is still with us. It comes from our families, our schools, advertising, and all the entertainment media. The old definition says being feminine means, among other things, waiting to be called for a date, waiting for a boy to open the car door for you, being a "good listener" and not expressing disagreement, never competing seriously with men for anything, and being mainly interested in "getting" a man. Slowly, though, more and more people are coming to understand that a woman is no less a woman when she opens her own car door, when she fights for what she deserves, when she feels comfortable expressing her opinions about things.

We've been told for a long time that men and women are different, and that is certainly true. We tend, for instance, to be more sensitive to other people's needs. And changing the definition of femininity doesn't mean that we need to give up that sensitivity. What changing the definition means is that we don't have to be sensitive to others *all* the time, even when it's against our own interests. And it can mean, too, that we don't think that men always have to look strong and in control. It can mean that men can learn to be more sensitive to others than they usually are.

Being feminine is often taken to mean not being competitive. Except, of course, when it comes to competing with other women for the prize of a man. When she's "out to get" a man, a woman is supposed to become hard and calculating and determined and stubborn. But if she's that way about getting a promotion or winning a game of tennis, there are people who'll say she's "unfeminine." Competitiveness is as much a part of a woman's nature as it is of a man's. But women are only supposed to express it in very narrow ways.

It's true that men and women differ physically. Men and women look different. Women are lighter on the average. Our chemical makeup is different from men's. And women usually live longer and are generally healthier all their lives than men. But thus far, there's very little evidence that what are called "feminine" traits are things that women are born with. Although typically masculine and feminine behavior shows up in very young children, that seems to be more the result of the way they're trained than it is of the way they're born. No one has yet proved that girls are born to be less intelligent, less aggressive, or more emotional than men.

What Can a Woman Do?

Certainly women are able to do whatever jobs are available to us. In our homes, we lift and carry and scrub, without giving it a second thought. The jobs we've had at times in our history have been jobs that are usually thought of as men's jobs. During World War II, women worked the farms and factories of this country. Employers provided day-care centers right at the workplace to make it convenient for mothers to work. And women performed at least as well as men did at the jobs they took. No one worried about a woman's being too unstable or emotional or weak to work; women were needed. When the men came back from the war, women were no longer needed in those jobs. Once again it was assumed that women were not able to do the same jobs as men and, besides, they should stay home and take care of husband, house, and kids. So women were laid off, the day-care centers were closed, and women gradually started again to believe the propaganda that said they were not only different from men but inferior as well.

But vast numbers of women have always worked in this country on farms, in textile mills, in factories, in offices, hospitals, and schools. Women usually work to support themselves and their families, not in order to have money for "luxuries." Women in this country are not encouraged to take themselves seriously as workers and wage earners, even though most women will work at some time in their lives, and many of us will work all of our adult lives.

If you ask a married man what he does, he's not likely to say, "I'm a husband and father, and I also work as a postman." Men usually identify themselves first by what they do. If you ask a woman what she does, she'll generally talk first about her domestic life as wife and mother, and only second about her outside job. We're expected to take our family responsibilities most seriously but, unfortunately, that sometimes makes it difficult or impossible for us to think seriously about careers. If you grow up believing that someone else is always going to support you, and that that's the way things should be, it's going to be hard for you to take your education seriously and to plan your working life so that it's the best it can be. If, instead, you assume that you'll have to work outside your home eventually, you can get a head start in thinking about and planning for what you really want to do.

Some time when you're unhappy about something, someone is bound to come along and tell you that you shouldn't be unhappy because these are *the best years of your life.* The person who tells you that is probably someone who doesn't remember her or his own teenage years very clearly. You're under all kinds of pressure to do and be different things. And a lot of the things that other people want you to be have very little to do with who *you* are.

There are probably lots of things that you'd like to do but can't, because of restrictions imposed on you by your parents, your school, your community, and the law. And there are probably things that you have to do that you hate. At every age of your life there are going to be restrictions on what you can do. While you're a teenager, though, you're expected to act like an adult a lot of the time, without getting many of the privileges that adults have. Add to this the fact that the demands and pressures on you are sometimes unreasonable, and that you're often not sure what to do about it, and you realize that you may sometimes have good cause to be unhappy.

Your life isn't all bad, though, and you know that. You do have fun, and you can have a sense that you're growing and trying new things. You have the freedom now to open up your thinking about what the rest of your life will be like. And you're living at a time when much of what was once taken for grant-ed about being a woman is being questioned and challenged.

It is possible (though still not easy) for you to do things that your mother never thought of doing, or to do things that she thought of but simply wasn't allowed to do, or to do without a fight things that your mother fought very hard for. You have new choices and new opportunities. They won't just fall into your lap. But they're there, if you really want them. There are probably too many people telling you what to do right now for these to be the *best* years of your life. But if you can get some understanding of who's telling you what and why—and, most important, if you can get some understanding of what *you* want and why—your chances of getting something positive out of these years will be much improved.

3

Girls and Girls

Most of us grow up believing that men are more important than women. Hardly anyone comes right out and says that, of course, but we do all seem to get the idea. When a boy is born, his family may start saving to send him to college. When a girl is born, her parents often figure, "She's just going to get married anyway, so why send her to college?" When a man is offered a job in a distant city, it's assumed that his wife will give up her job, her friends, and her family contacts and go with him. When one member of a couple has to work to put the other through school, it's almost always the woman who postpones or gives up her education so that the man can get his. And if you had been planning to spend an evening with your girlfriend and a boy calls to ask you out, the chances are that you won't think twice about canceling out on your girlfriend.

From the time a girl is born, many people assume that the crowning achievement of her life will be "getting a man." She's encouraged to flirt when she's still a baby. Her Barbie doll has a boyfriend, so that while a girl is still little, she can act out dating and marriage fantasies. Then, when a girl gets to be a teenager, the pressure really goes on. Boys become more and more important in her life—or at least they're *supposed* to be important, if you believe what you read and hear. Girls are constantly bombarded with books about how to get boyfriends, and every girls' magazine has at least one article on the subject every month. And meanwhile, so little attention is paid to friendships between girls that you could easily get the idea that they are not important. But the friendships you form with other girls are among the most valuable relationships you can have.

Much too often, you'll hear a woman say, "I really like men better than I like women," or, "I really can't stand women." For a woman to say that probably means not only that she thinks other women are inferior to men, but that she thinks she's inferior too. She's saying that a woman can't be interesting or likable or just nice to be with. If you can't find any reasons to like other women, you'll not only have a hard time liking yourself, but you'll miss out on the friendships you could have with half the people around you.

Women versus Women

If you never question the idea that getting a man is the most important thing for a woman, then it becomes easy for you to put down other women, and even to make all other women your enemies (since you can only see them as competition for men). Everyone in this society is taught to compete. But boys are allowed to compete openly—in sports or in school or simply by fighting with one another. Since a girl's goal is supposed to be to catch a man, she often has no way to compete with other women except to achieve that goal.

The kind of open competition that men have doesn't have to destroy their friendships. (Many men have a hard time establishing close friendships, but that's because they can't express their feelings openly, not because of competition between them.) You can probably imagine two boys having a knock-down-drag-out fight over a girl and still being friends. But girls usually don't have fights over boys. Many girls plot and plan all sorts of schemes to get or keep boyfriends. And all that plotting can easily keep you from getting too close to other girls. It can poison friendships that already exist, or it can keep you from making friends with a girl because you're afraid that she really wants to steal your boyfriend. Some girls (probably most girls at one time or another) get so wrapped up in getting a boyfriend (or keeping one) that they do things that they *know* are inexcusable. If you let yourself get totally involved in catching and keeping a boyfriend, it's easy to do things to your friends that you otherwise wouldn't think of doing—like lying to them or about them or backstabbing.

A Girl Can Be Your Best Friend

In spite of the fact that a lot less energy seems to go into friendships with girls than goes into keeping boyfriends, those friendships continue to be formed and often last a lifetime. At a time in your life when you may often feel uncomfortable and unsure of yourself with a boy, a friendship with another girl can give you an opportunity to relax and learn to express your feelings. You don't have to worry about whether you should call her up; there's no one saying that you have to wait for *her* to call *you*. You don't have to feel uncertain about telling another girl what *you* want to do. And, once you get started, it's usually easier to talk to another girl about your real feelings.

There's still likely to be a tendency to say things to your girlfriend that you think she wants to hear or will agree with. If you have thoughts or feelings that you think she may not share, you may be afraid to talk about them because you don't want her to think you're peculiar. Most teenagers seem to have the idea that everyone around knows something that they themselves don't know. Everyone else looks and acts very cool. Though you may try to act as cool as the others, you know that underneath it all you're insecure and unsure of what to do. What's really going on is that everyone is walking around feeling the same way you do, though that may be hard for you to believe. In fact, there are people who live out their lives feeling that they never know quite how to act or what to say and that everyone else does. All those cool-looking people don't really know some secret you don't. You have to believe you look as cool to other people as they look to you.

The feelings of unsureness that you have can be terribly hard to talk about, since no one else seems to want to admit that she has them too. Or at least no one wants to be the *first* to admit to them. If you have a girlfriend with whom you feel comfortable, though, that's the place to start talking. It's an immense relief to learn that you're not alone in the way you feel.

It's frightening sometimes even to think about admitting to someone else how different you feel. What you expect (and fear) is that she's going to say, "Oh, I don't feel that way at all." And then you'll be left exposed, having admitted that you're not as cool and sure of yourself as you'd like to be. But what probably will happen is that once you've opened up, your friend will get the courage to talk about her own feelings, which will turn out to be not so different from yours. Hard as it may be for you to talk with someone else about how you really feel, you may find it easier in the long run than always having to keep your image propped up. And once you've managed to relax and open up with one person, you may find that it's then easier with others.

You may be afraid of opening up to a friend and having her use what you've said against you somehow. That does happen occasionally. The best insur-

ance against that is to choose your friend carefully.
If you believe you can trust someone, the chances
are you're right. And if for some reason you feel you
cannot trust someone, the chances are you're right
about that too. Don't pick someone who's known to
gossip; don't pick someone who's told you someone
else's secrets. She's bound to repeat yours as well.

People may sometimes advise you never to confide your deepest feelings to anyone because of the
risk of having your confidences used against you.
But it really is worth the risk. You don't have to spill
everything all at once anyway, and the friend who
keeps a little secret is likely to keep a big one too.
You probably already have some idea which of your
friends you can trust and which you can't because of
things that have already happened. You can test your
own judgment about others slowly and carefully,
gradually learning to trust others and to trust your
judgments about them.

Girlfriends versus Boyfriends

If you get very involved with a boy, you may let
your friendships with girls lapse and only pick them
up again when you and the boy break up. The boyfriend seems more "important" somehow. But in
fact your girlfriends are probably the ones with
whom you're able to be more comfortable, more
open, more really yourself. If you stop having anything to do with your old friends just because you're

involved with a boy, you shouldn't expect them to still be there when you and your boyfriend break up. If you don't call your "best" girlfriend for six months, and then you want her to be there because you need a shoulder to cry on, don't expect her to act too generous. You've treated her shabbily and you shouldn't expect anything better in return.

If you choose your friends because you like them and you are comfortable with them, then your friendships are more valuable to you in the long run than a passing romance, although the romance may be a good deal more intense for a while. Your friends shouldn't be let go when it's convenient for you and picked up when you have nowhere else to go. You have to keep in mind that a close friend or group of friends will get you through times when you don't have a boyfriend better than a boyfriend will get you through times when you don't have any other friends at all. It may take a special effort on your part to keep up your friendships when you're very much emotionally involved with someone, but it's worthwhile.

Between Girls

Sometimes when you develop a particularly close relationship with another girl you may find that you have sexual feelings and sexual fantasies about her. Like any other new and strong feelings, these can be frightening. Besides, a lot of people have been taught that having sexual feelings toward a person of the same sex means that you are weird or sick. You may have heard the word "lesbian" and wonder if you are one.

First, be assured that sexual feelings between girls are *very* common. Most women have them at some time in their lives. So stop thinking that you're peculiar. Trying to deny, especially to yourself, that you have these feelings is not a good way to deal with them. If they exist, you might as well acknowledge that they're there and try to learn something from them. For many girls, the first conscious sexual feelings that they have for another person involve another girl or a woman. Even if you don't act on your feelings, you've learned that you can be sexually attracted to another human being, which is a good thing to know about yourself.

A great many women have a sexual *experience* with another woman at some time in their lives. So that's not very rare either. What does it mean for you if you do have a sexual experience with another girl? It doesn't necessarily mean that you can't or won't also have sexual feelings for boys. It can mean that you have had a sexual experience from which you've learned something about your feelings and about your body, how it functions, and what gives you pleasure. It can strengthen or destroy a relationship. There's no right or wrong about sexual feelings or actions, unless someone is being forced to do something she doesn't want to do. If either of you doesn't want the experience and feels forced into it, or if either of you feels strong shame or guilt, the effect on your relationship will be bad. That applies to relations with the same sex and relations with the opposite sex equally well. But if you can take your experiences with your friend (or your feelings or your fantasies) as a normal part of growing up, you can learn some good things about yourself.

Some women choose to relate sexually only to other women, and these women are called lesbians. You may find yourself among them, if you decide that you prefer sexual relationships with women over sexual relationships with men. The percentage of women (or men, for that matter) who are exclusively homosexual all their lives is actually quite small, much smaller than the percentage who've had one or a few homosexual experiences. Some people are *homosexual* (they relate to people of the same sex) when they're young and are *heterosexual* (they relate to people of the opposite sex) when they're older. People who have the ability to relate sexually to both men and women are called *bisexuals.* Some people are heterosexual for years and then become homosexual. If we weren't taught that there is something wrong with being homosexual, more people might choose to have homosexual relationships all or part of the time.

If you find that you would like a place to talk about your homosexual feelings and experiences, and you don't have a sympathetic friend or adult to talk to, you'll have to face the fact that finding an understanding listener may be difficult. There are gay groups in most big cities, many smaller cities and towns, and on many college campuses (even in a few high schools), and most of these groups are happy to provide support and counseling for young people. Most of them will be able to help you find out what you want to know, but there's always the possibility that you could run into a group whose concern is more with convincing you to be gay than with helping you individually. Or you may find, if you talk with a friend or an adult you thought sympathetic, or even with a psychiatrist, that his or her concern is more with convincing you not to be gay. Just remember that, whomever you talk to, you'll still have to make your own decisions based on what's best for you.

The Group

Whatever your problems as a teenager are, one of the ways you can share your problems and feelings and maybe get some help with them is to get together to talk with a small group of girls. You can learn that you're not alone, that most of the girls in the group are working on solving the same problems that you are. And you can help one another. You can talk about the kinds of problems you have with your parents and try to find ways to handle them better. You can find out how one person coped with being gossiped about or how another told her steady boy-friend that she wanted to date other people.

You'll also find in a group that there are things that you've got worked out that other people haven't. In those areas, you can help them to grow, just as in others they can help you. You learn that mistakes, yours and other people's, are as important as successes, because you can all learn from your own and one another's mistakes. That way, each of you doesn't have to learn everything alone by trial and error.

Whether you are going to be talking to one friend or to a group, the important things that develop between friends are trust and support. You have to be ready to be honest; to be able to accept another person as she is with all her faults and weaknesses; to be happy for her, not jealous, when good things happen to her; to be helpful, patient, and sympathetic when bad things happen; and not to talk to others about the things she's told you.

That's a great deal to ask of yourself. But since that's what you would want from a friend, that's what you have to be prepared to give. Your friendships are worth the effort, since they are relationships in which you can grow, learn to be yourself, and learn a lot about who you really are. A friend who likes some (not necessarily all) of the things that you do, whom you like to be with, whom you can really talk to, can be your friend all your life.

4

Girls and Boys

You've probably noticed that teenage girls are often judged according to who their boyfriends are. The girl who goes out with the most popular boy in school is automatically popular and desirable. And the girl who goes out with a boy who's fat or not good-looking or who doesn't have a car or who's just not very popular often feels uncomfortable being seen with him, because she thinks people will wonder what's wrong with her. However, in neither case does her choice of a boyfriend necessarily tell you anything about who a girl really is. The popular boy may be nice, or he may be a complete creep; the same goes for the unpopular boy. And the girl who goes with a popular boy doesn't automatically have a happier life in the long run than the girl who goes out with the class weirdo.

Nevertheless, most teenage girls spend a good part of their time worrying about boys. If you don't have a boyfriend, you may think it's because there's something wrong with you. If you do have a boyfriend, then you may spend your time worrying about him and your relationship and your feelings and his feelings and how you're supposed to act. If you just happen to be the most popular girl in your school and the head of the cheerleading squad *and* you're going steady with the captain of the football team, you still probably spend as much time worrying about boys as anyone else. If you go steady, you probably sometimes envy the girls who get to go out with lots of guys; and if you don't have a steady, you may wish that you did. And finally, if you're one of the many girls who hardly ever dates or never dates at all, you may feel that you're the only girl in the world who doesn't have dates all the time, even though most girls go through periods when they don't date very much.

Getting a date or a boyfriend sometimes becomes so important to a girl that she loses her whole sense of proportion about it. It's not hard to understand why this happens. Everything seems to give you the idea that getting a boyfriend *is* the most important thing you can do; that getting a boyfriend will make you happy, solve all your problems, improve your disposition, clear up your acne; and that you'll know exactly how to act when you do get one. No one comes right out and *says* those things, but they're implied. So in the race to get a boyfriend, you can not only neglect the rest of your life (your girlfriends, your other interests, etc.), but you may find that you're not really caring about *who* the boy is— just so long as he's a boy.

Everyone seems to realize that relationships between teenage girls and teenage boys can be difficult, but it's not surprising that you may very much want to have a boyfriend anyway. There may be places you can't go or places where you'd feel uncomfortable without a date. So if you don't have a boy to go with, you may feel miserable and left out of things. You may feel embarrassed about not having a date or a steady boyfriend. If you feel unhappy about not having a boyfriend, it will probably help if you admit that to yourself and maybe also to your friends, instead of going around trying to look like you just don't care. Have a good cry about it if you want to, find something else to do, and try to remember that having a boyfriend doesn't make you a better person. And not having a boyfriend doesn't mean that boys don't like you, or that you're unattractive, or that your life is a failure.

What's Going On in His Head?

Boys, while they're teenagers, are going through many of the same changes that girls are. They are growing up, learning about themselves and other people, thinking about the future. And they are having as hard a time as you figuring out who they are. However, boys have some additional problems. Since being masculine (to many people) means being tough and cool and aggressive, it's considered even less acceptable for a boy to look unsure of himself than it is for a girl. And boys are usually taught not to show their emotions ("Big boys don't cry"), so it's sometimes terribly difficult for them to express their feelings at all, even when they know what those feelings are. Very often, though, boys really don't know how they feel about things.

A lot of boys just can't measure up to what's expected of them. Hopefully, by the time a boy grows up, he'll be able to give up trying to look tough and cool and aggressive *all* the time. But as a teenager, a boy may feel that he has to try to live up to that image. A man, of course, isn't necessarily strong and unemotional just because he's a man, any more than a woman is necessarily weak and warm and emotional just because she's a woman. But the pressure on a boy to act "manly" can make him lose touch with his real feelings completely. He can spend so much time and energy trying to look the way he's told to be that he eventually forgets he doesn't always feel that way at all.

You've probably heard that teenage girls are more "mature" than teenage boys. It's true that teenage girls, on the whole, handle relations with other people better than boys do. So some of the problems that girls have with boys stem from that fact alone. You may be ready for a serious relationship sooner than he is. You may be more able to make a good decision about whom to have a relationship with, while underneath his cool, he's probably shyer and less sure of himself than you are. Two boys (or two men) can be friends for years without ever having a serious talk about themselves and their feelings. It may only be because girls and women are encouraged to be more open about our feelings, but we are generally better able to recognize what our feelings are and deal with them than are men.

Do You Go Out and Who With?

There are some circumstances where you can feel better about yourself if you don't have a boyfriend than if you do. For instance, if the boy who asks you out is someone you really don't like, or someone who makes you uncomfortable, you'll probably have a miserable time if you go out with him. If his only interests are things you don't like, you're better off without him and he without you. And if the boy who asks you out is your girlfriend's boyfriend, you may have to decide between having a date (realizing that he may be taking you out *only* because he's trying to make her jealous) and having a friend. Since friendships last longer than dates, the choice seems clear. In any case, you have to make a decision about what's really important to you and what isn't.

If a boy asks you out and you have no intention of going out with him, that time or ever, the best thing you can do is make that clear by saying, as kindly as you can, "I'm sorry, but I don't want to go out with you." That's not an easy thing to say to anyone, but putting him off by saying, "Maybe another time," or by giving him excuses is just plain unfair. Saying no firmly and definitely is the hardest thing to do in the short run, but in the long run it's kinder to the boy than leading him on by never giving him a straight answer.

You don't have to limit yourself to going out only with boys that you're in love with. You can have casual dates or a long, close relationship with a boy that you like but don't love. It may be more satisfying for you to see a lot of someone with whom you can be relaxed because the emotional involvement isn't very heavy. You'll probably be able to be more open with him and to learn a lot about boys from him, too.

Keeping Him in Perspective

If you're going out with someone, and you're thinking about going steady, you have to look closely at *why* you want to go steady with him. The advantage, of course, is that you're always sure of having a date when you want one. The disadvantage to going steady is that it may limit the number and kinds of experiences you can have. One boy can't possibly fulfill all of your needs. Even if you don't date others, you need to have other friends—of both sexes. And you may find that you want to have dates with more than one person. You may be most interested in one boy, and like him best, but still want less intense relationships with others.

Once you have a boyfriend, especially a steady boyfriend, his friends often become your friends. That's fine as long as his friends don't become your only friends. What usually happens is that you tend to do things with *his* friends and *their* girlfriends, not with *your* friends and *their* boyfriends. But your friends, the ones *you* choose, are a better reflection of your *self* and who you really are than your boyfriend's friends are.

As a rule, it is the boy you're going out with who decides what you'll do and who you'll do it with. So if your best friend doesn't have a boyfriend, or if her boyfriend and yours aren't already friends, she probably won't be included in your social life unless you make a special effort to have her included (and hope she does the same for you).

When you're going out with someone, you may find that you always agree to see the movies *he* likes or to do the things *he* wants to do. You may find that you either pretend to agree with his opinions or that you just don't disagree openly with him (even when you know he's wrong about something). You may find that you're afraid to say anything when you're bored with whatever you're doing, because you're afraid he won't ask you out again.

If he's doing something you don't like, or if you're bored to death, you might as well let him know. That doesn't mean you shouldn't sometimes listen when

he's talking about things that don't especially interest you (you might even *get* interested), or that he
always has to take you where you want to go, even if
it doesn't interest him. But a lot of boys assume that
they'll always make decisions about what to do and
where to go, and a lot of girls never stop to question
that. There's no reason for you to always put his
feelings before yours. If he never wants to do or talk
about things that *you* want to do or talk about, then
you're not getting much out of the relationship. In
that case, it's not the end of the world if he doesn't
ask you out again. And if he likes you, he's not going
to end the relationship because you don't always go
along with what he wants or thinks. He shouldn't be
afraid to let you make decisions too. And besides, if
you always let him make the decisions, you're never
going to learn to make them for yourself.

Rules and How to Break Them

Girls are often told that it's very important not to
threaten a boy's ego, never to let him know how
much you know or how well you can do something.
You're told, for instance, that if you play Ping-Pong
better than he does, you shouldn't beat him at it,
because that will make him feel bad. But if you *can*
beat him at Ping-Pong and you *don't* (or if you don't
let him know that you know more about cars or
cooking or football or whatever), you're not being
honest and you're not being yourself. Teasing him

about being a lousy Ping-Pong player or for not knowing about something isn't called for, however. In any relationship, whether with a boy or a girl, there's no excuse for rubbing in someone else's weaknesses.

There are lots of rules about relating to boys that are supposed to make it easier for everyone to know how to act, but a lot of those rules just get in the way. You can open doors for yourself. You can even hold a door open for someone else, male or female, if they're carrying something or if you happen to get to the door first. It's an awfully uncomfortable, even silly, situation when you get to the door first and then wait for a boy to reach around you to get it open while you just stand there. It takes years of practice for most boys until they can do that one gracefully, and most of them would be just as happy not to have to try. And if you open the door yourself, you don't have to stand there wondering whether or not he'll remember to open it or whether he's going to step on your feet trying.

If you want to call a boy on the phone, whether it's just because you want to talk or whether there's really something you have to ask him that no one else knows, then you should call him. Some boys, unfortunately, can't deal with being called by a girl since they're very concerned about being the one who does the calling. So you'll have to use your judgment. If you have a feeling that he's the kind of boy who's going to be totally turned off to you if you call him, then you'd better not, unless you can think up a really good excuse. On the other hand, there are a lot of boys who'd be happy not to always have to call you. And if he's shy, he may just be delighted to have you make the first move. Of course, if he *never* calls you back, or never wants to talk when you call, you should be able to get the message that he's not interested. You still haven't lost anything, though. If he does like you, he's not going to stop liking you just because you call him. And if you weren't sure whether or not he liked you, at least you've given him an opening and given yourself a chance to find out.

You can also ask a boy for a date. Here again, you have to use your judgment about how the boy will react. And you have to risk being turned down. Boys take that risk all the time when they ask girls out, and they all seem to survive, so you will too. You may feel most comfortable asking him to a turn-around party or to a party being given by a friend of yours that he wouldn't otherwise go to. Or you could give a party just to have an excuse to ask him, if you want to give a party. Or you can ask him to go swimming or bowling or to the movies or a concert with a group, which isn't quite so much like a "date." You can ask a boy out, and he may be as pleased and flattered as you are when someone asks you out.

And that brings us to the question of who pays for a date. If the boy always pays for your dates, he may feel that it's his right to decide what you're going to do. And, as a matter of fact, there's a certain logic to his feeling that way, since he *is* the one who's paying. In this country, it's a pretty well established custom that the man pays. But there are countries in Europe, for example, where it's unheard of for a teenage girl not to pay for herself when she goes out with someone. There are a couple of advantages to paying your own way, at least once in a while. It can make it easier for you to suggest doing what you want to do. It can help you understand that you don't have to be grateful for being asked out. (Not that you should have to feel grateful anyway. If a boy asks you out, it's because he wants to be with you. So, by simply being there, you've fulfilled your end of the deal.) The boy may also appreciate your paying for yourself, since that may make it possible for you both to do things that he couldn't afford to pay for alone.

There may be some problems about paying your own way. Just as older women with jobs almost always earn less than men (for the same work), teenage girls generally earn less from odd jobs than teenage boys. If both of you get an allowance, his may well be larger than yours. Either way, it's possible that he has more money to spend than you do. Or you may need your money for other things. So it may be a real financial hardship for you to pay for a date.

Some teenage boys will unfortunately feel that their masculinity is being questioned if you offer to pay. That's ridiculous, of course, since masculinity has nothing to do with money, but he may not have figured that out yet. It can't hurt, though, to suggest that you sometimes pay for yourself, if you want to. It's not going to end what would otherwise have been the all-time beautiful relationship. And he might really like the arrangement. You might also try to find some things to do that don't cost money, which gets you around the whole problem.

Some girls like to invite a boy to their house for an evening, which is one of those things to do that don't cost money. You might feel comfortable about doing that or you might not. If you live in a small house or apartment where everyone's always on top of everyone else, you may not like having friends over. Most teenage boys would rather go through the fires of hell than spend an evening in the same room with a girl's parents. Or you may know that there's no threat or bribe that will keep your little brother from being in the way. Or you may just prefer to keep your social life and your family life separate. If spending an evening at home with a boy means that you're going to be teased unmercifully by your entire family for weeks afterward, then you'll probably feel (and rightly so) that it's not worth it.

"Getting Involved" and "Falling in Love"

It's not particularly good for you to let your life get centered on one person, but it can be easier to do that than you expect. The feelings you may have in a relationship with a boy can sometimes be overpowering. And when you're having those feelings, especially the first time, they can be difficult to deal with. You may find that you think about nothing but HIM. You spend as much time as you can daydreaming about him. You make complicated plans for "unexpectedly" running into him. Unless you're actually with him or talking on the phone, you're always waiting for him to call or to arrive. You may lose your appetite and find that you can't concentrate on your schoolwork or anything else that doesn't have to do with him. You cover pages in your notebook with his name. You don't make plans to do anything, just in case he calls.

Fortunately, this stage usually doesn't last too long. If you are actually having a relationship with this wonderful creature, your feelings should eventually settle down enough so that you can go on with your own life. If he doesn't know that you're alive (or if he knows but doesn't care, which is worse), you may have a harder time. If you never have any real contact with him, you never find out about his failings and you can continue to dream that he's perfect, which will make him harder to get over.

In any case, you should try to keep yourself together as much as possible. If you're having a relationship, try to keep it a *part* of your life. That means keeping up with all the things you usually do and continuing to spend time with your other friends. If you're not having a relationship, and if it looks like the boy is not going to get interested in you, then you not only have to keep your life going, but you have to try to talk yourself out of your feelings. You *can* do that, if you want to enough, though it's easier said than done.

The first time you fall in love is really different from any other time, simply because you've never done it before. You don't know yet how to express your feelings, or if you should express them, or how to act when you're with him. You may feel so good (or so bad, if your love isn't returned) that you can't believe this ever happened to anyone before.

The first time you love someone (other than your family or friends, which is a different kind of love), you will probably feel very sure that it's going to last forever. You might (though the chances are slim) continue to love your first love for the rest of your life. Even if you do, the kind of love and the strength of your feelings will continue to change as you change. If your feelings change so that you're less attached to your first love as time goes on, that's all right too. It doesn't mean that you didn't really love him. It simply means that, as you have changed and grown, your needs have changed and he no longer fills them; or that, as he has changed and grown, he has become a different person from the one you fell in love with. Love doesn't have to last forever in order to be "real love."

When you fall in love with someone, you have to keep in mind that he is still the same person he was before you loved him. Your love won't make him perfect. He has good and bad points, and you have to accept those as much as you can, just as you hope he'll be able to accept yours. You can't expect to change him. If he is unhappy with something about himself, and if he wants to change that, he has to do it himself. You can't make him change, and you can't do it for him. You can help, by being frank about things that displease you. And since he's not perfect, there will be things about him that displease you. But you have to be ready to put up with those things until and unless he's ready to do something about them.

Just as you can't make someone change, you can't make someone love you. You can (and probably should) try to get him to notice that you're there since, if he doesn't know that, you haven't got a chance for a relationship. But people love others out of their own feelings, and you can't force him to have feelings he doesn't have. If he doesn't love you to begin with, he's not going to love you just because you sleep with him or do his math homework for him. You also can't prove to someone that you love him by doing something for him. He either believes it or he doesn't (and if you say you love him, why shouldn't he believe it?), and doing something for him won't change that.

Love can grow in a relationship, and the fact that you don't love each other "at first sight" doesn't mean you won't love each other later. The growth of love is based on a whole lot of things—getting to know someone, learning to trust him, sharing experiences, and gradually becoming close. Love grows over a period of time, and not all at once, though you can be very attracted to someone the first time you meet him.

How can you be sure that you love someone? I don't know that you *can* be sure. There have been millions of definitions of "love," and some of them might apply to the way you feel and some might not. Whether you love someone or not isn't determined by how long your feelings last. It's determined by how strong your feelings are, how much you care for that person, not whether the feelings last for six days or sixty years. Since you can never predict exactly what's going to happen in a relationship (although sometimes you have an idea whether things are going to be good or bad), it might be best for you to consider yourself in love when you *think* you're in love. Lots and lots of people love each other, get married, and then stop loving each other and get divorced, and no one assumes that they didn't really love each other to begin with. If you feel like you love someone, then the definitions of love hardly matter, and you might as well take your feelings seriously.

What to Do When You Don't Get Along

A relationship with someone you love isn't perfect. It's in fairy tales, and *only* in fairy tales, that people live "happily ever after." The romantic dreams of "becoming one," of never fighting, never being unhappy with each other, never disagreeing about anything, are dreams and stories—they're not real. Real people who love each other can and do have fights and disagreements without destroying their relationship. Being angry with someone doesn't mean that you don't love him. And letting your anger out is better for you and for the relationship than trying to pretend it isn't there. With any strong feelings, you can't just make them go away. So your anger is going to come out somehow. If you're angry with someone you love (or someone you don't love, for that matter), you don't have to jump up and down and scream and yell, though you can do that too, if that's what you feel like doing. But if you're afraid to show your anger, you can at least say calmly to the other person, "Look, I'm really furious about ————." After a while, it gets easier to express anger as you learn that getting angry doesn't have to mean the end of the relationship. And if the other person can't deal with your anger, either he will have to change or you should find yourself someone who can.

There are a couple of rules for constructive arguing that you should try to stick to. The first is to try, no matter how angry you are and no matter how loud you yell, to stick to the issue and not attack the person. *Don't* tell him he's stupid and he can't do *anything* right. By doing that, you're attacking who he is. Stick to attacking what he's *done*. If he's always late and waiting is driving you crazy, tell him *that*. The second rule is not to put up with physical violence. There is absolutely no reason in the world to let him knock you around because he happens to be stronger, or vice versa. And finally, you also have to give the other person the space to be angry with you, without assuming that because he's angry about something you've done, he doesn't love you anymore.

What Can Go Wrong?

There are a number of things that will destroy any relationship. One is dishonesty, whether on your part or his. You may both feel perfectly happy dating several different people and find that that doesn't hurt your relationship a bit. But if you're supposed to be going steady, and you're not going out with anyone else, and you find out that the boy *has* been, then you have every right to be angry and hurt. Talk to him and tell him what you know. If he denies it, that means he's not about to change, and you are going to have to get out of the relationship. If he promises to stop, give him the chance. If he promises to stop and doesn't, then you really are better off without him, because he's not to be trusted.

Jealousy can be completely destructive to a relationship, especially when it isn't based on any reality. If every time you see him talking to another girl, you assume that he's two-timing you, or if you assume when he doesn't call that it's because he's with someone else, then you really have a problem. Sometimes you get involved with a boy who does that sort of thing to you, who constantly tries to make you account for every minute that you don't spend with him, or who accuses you of flirting if you talk to another boy. That kind of jealousy is usually a sign that the person is so unsure of himself that he can't accept the fact that someone really likes him. However, whatever its cause, it's unbearable for the other person, who feels suffocated by it. If you're suffering from this kind of jealousy (and it *is* suffering), try, if you can, not to let the boy know that you're so jealous. Questioning him, when he's innocent, will probably make him furious and drive him away. If he continues to pay attention to you, that should be enough to convince you that he really does like you. Instead of talking to him about your problem, try talking to a friend who knows both of you and may be able to give the support and reassurance you need. Getting another person's view of the relationship will help you see it more clearly yourself.

Another of the things that can destroy a relationship is guilt. Guilt can arise around sex, or it can come from things like seeing someone on the sly because your parents don't approve of him, or letting yourself get involved in things that you'd rather not do. None of which *has* to produce guilt, of course. But if you are doing something that makes you feel guilty, eventually you're probably going to blame the boy for your guilt, and you can wind up hating him. The only solution is not to do something if you know beforehand that you're going to feel guilty about it afterward. And if you do something that you didn't think you'd feel guilty about, but you find that you do anyway, then you have to avoid doing it again. None of this is easy.

Letting yourself be taken advantage of or letting yourself be treated badly will also probably lead to your hating the boy, as well as to not feeling too happy with yourself. That's not to say that you have to go by anyone else's rules about what's good treatment and what's not. If he has a habit of calling you in the afternoon when he wants to see you that evening, and if that doesn't bother you, then there's no problem and no reason to insist on another arrangement. If you can go ahead and make plans (and stick to them) whether he calls or not, then you aren't wasting your life sitting by the telephone. However, if you find that you never make plans to do anything on your own because you're hoping he'll call at the last minute, then you're hanging yourself up. Eventually, you're going to start resenting the fact that you're always waiting around. If he's making your life miserable by always keeping you waiting, or purposely making you jealous, or putting you down in public or in private, or making demands that you don't want to meet, you've got yourself in a bad relationship.

Your friends or your parents may think your boyfriend is terrific, but if the relationship you have with him doesn't satisfy you, then you're better off without him. And if you have a relationship that makes *you* happy, but the boy isn't popular with your friends, then trust your own judgment. The test of a relationship is how it makes you feel, not whether it meets someone else's idea of what the perfect relationship should be.

Mr. Wrong

Almost every woman, it seems, falls in love at some time in her life with a man who's really wrong for her. Sometimes he's a man she really doesn't *like*; or he might be someone who is inappropriate, like someone else's boyfriend or husband. These attractions can be terribly strong—much too strong for most of us simply to do what would be best, which is to forget all about him. So if you get yourself into one of these relationships (and you'll know it's a wrong one if it comes along), you'll eventually have to get yourself out, for the sake of your sanity and your self-respect. Unfortunately there's no fast or easy way out. There is one thing, though, that you can try which will almost certainly work, given enough time. It may take a year or more, but it's worth trying. What you have to do is to think as positively as possible about yourself. You *know* you deserve a better relationship than you've got; so keep reminding yourself of that. Develop the things

that you do best. Work on improving other relationships, go out with other people whenever you can,
and keep telling yourself that you *should* have good
relationships with people.

While you're being positive about yourself, you
have to think negatively about the relationship.
Make a list of everything you like about yourself and
know you can do well. Then make a list of everything that's wrong with the relationship. Then,
whenever you think about him, try to think of something positive about yourself and something negative about the relationship. It may take a while, but
you should eventually get to the point where he no
longer seems so desirable.

If you always seem to get involved with boys who
treat you badly, you have a more serious problem.
The problem then is that you *don't* believe that you
deserve better. A lot of times there's even a nice guy
around whom you like and who likes you, but he
just doesn't excite you. And you only get really involved with the boys who excite you, who happen to
be the ones who aren't nice to you. Sometimes you
can get out of this pattern by yourself. Sometimes
you just outgrow it. You get into bad relationships
because you sense that they *won't* last forever, so
they're safe in a way. Then when you're ready for a
serious involvement, you choose someone you can
really care about. What has happened is that you've
learned to like yourself and learned that you're
worth something. But if you keep having bad rela-

tionships—and there are women who *marry* a series of terrible men—then you might think about getting psychological counseling or therapy to help you break the pattern.

One bad relationship doesn't necessarily mean that you'll have others, or that you should immediately get professional help. Most women seem to have at least one attractive creep in their past. If you can learn something from the relationship (like what you *cannot* tolerate), you'll have made progress.

Breaking Up

Breaking up a relationship is usually painful for at least one of you. If you are the one doing the breaking up, try to make it as painless as possible for the other person. You may find that you feel guilty about hurting another person, but if you no longer care for him, it's obviously kinder to end the relationship sooner rather than later. If he does the breaking up, try to take the news with as much dignity as possible. There are times when you can't help but burst into tears, but don't try to use tears to hold on to him. Usually when someone's decided to break up, he means it and, though you may talk him into changing his mind for a while, sooner or later he'll try again.

Breaking up is often a terrible experience. At first, you may feel rejected and abandoned, and you may think you'll never be able to love or trust anyone ever again. You'll eventually start to feel better, although that's hard to believe at first. For a while, try to think more about what was bad about the relationship than about the good times you had. Try not to blame yourself for the breakup. Everyone makes mistakes in relationships, and he certainly must have made as many as you did. All you can do is determine not to make the same mistakes in your next relationship (though you'll probably make some of the same ones and some new ones as well). And, though it's hard to believe at first, there *will* be another relationship.

What's Most Important?

In any relationship, whether with a boy or a girl, you have to be able to feel comfortable. If you're constantly on your guard about saying or doing the wrong thing, if you can't express your feelings or your opinions, you're not getting much from the relationship in terms of your own needs and your own growth. If you find that you always have to act the way someone else wants you to, you'll eventually find that you don't even know how you *want* to behave. You'll have lost ground in learning who you really are by trying to act like someone you're not. Having a relationship with a boy who makes you unhappy, uncomfortable, or bored just isn't worth it. If you're not happy with the relationship you have, you have to change it or get out, either of which takes time.

No one always does exactly what she wants to do. In any relationship there are compromises to be made. But to compromise on one particular point (like whether to go to the beach or to the movies) and to compromise yourself on your basic needs or values are different things. You have to make as clear a decision as you can about what's really important to you, so that you know where you can give ground, what things you can be flexible about, and what things are too important to you to change your mind about.

Marriage

Many girls think of marriage simply as living with someone you love, who will love you and take care of you. You think about weddings and plan your own. You think of living in a nice little house or apartment, fixing intimate dinners for two, having your friends over, being able to do all the things you want to do. If you think about having children, you may think about happy, gurgling babies dressed up in cute clothes.

The reality of marriage is not much like most people's fantasies about it. Think about how you get along with the people you live with—your mother and father, sisters and brothers. You and your family, no matter how many differences there may be among you, share a history, habits, tastes, ways of doing and thinking about things. You and your husband, coming from different families, are going to have less in common. You can judge from looking at your own behavior at home just how well you'll be able to cope with the differences between you.

Living with another person always takes a certain amount of adjustment and compromise—from *both* parties. It's impossible to know what it's going to be like to live with someone until you've actually done it, but there are clues that you can look at. Does he have habits that bother you a little or a lot? How will you feel about those habits when you have to live with them? Does he know how to take care of himself, or does his mother make his bed, wash his clothes, and fix his lunch? Will he expect you to do all those things? Do you want to? If you don't want to, who will?

Conflicts in marriage arise from all sorts of things. If you come from a family where food isn't considered important, where dinner is usually a TV dinner out of the freezer, and he comes from a family where dinner is five courses with dessert, you're going to have to come to a compromise about meals that *both* of you can live with. If he wants kids right away and you don't because you want to work full time outside your home, you'll have to come to an understanding. And it's best done *before* you're married. Whatever the disagreement, resentment can build if one of you simply gives in to something without really agreeing with it. If you simply say, "Okay, I'll give up my job and have a baby," when you don't want a baby, how will you feel later? Will you wind up resenting both your husband (who "made" you have the baby) and the baby, because you'd rather be doing something else than taking care of it?

Whether you're thinking of getting married now or twenty years from now, there are some questions you'll want the answers to before you get married. Can you live with his basic values, even if they're not the same as yours? For instance, having the same religious background isn't important if neither of you is religious. But if religious practice is important to one or both of you, then differences about religion do have to be taken into consideration. Do you find his religion offensive? Or vice versa? Would it upset you if you had children and they were raised in his religion? You don't have to be the *same* when it comes to religion or background or values or life-styles, but you do have to be able to live with each other.

Do you agree about what men's and women's roles in marriage should be? Does he expect you to stay home and work full time taking care of the house and kids (or to work full time outside and take care of the house too) while he works outside and does nothing at home? Are you going to be happy with that? For twenty-plus years? How does he feel about doing housework? Does he think it's "women's work"? Do you?

The subjects of sharing housework and of women working outside the home have become sources of tremendous conflicts for many couples recently, and the two of you will probably have to deal with them eventually. Since attitudes on these subjects reflect some of people's most basic ideas about what it means to be a man or woman, it's a good idea to talk about them *before* you marry someone.

Take a look at the way disagreements between you are settled. Does he always insist on having his way? Do *you* always insist on having yours? Are both of you willing to listen to the other, respect the other's needs, and compromise? Do you think that two people can have a successful relationship when, over many years, *one* of them wins *all* the arguments?

Does he treat you as his equal? Does he expect you to be his mother or his daughter or his maid? How does he feel about your spending time away from him with your own friends? You don't have to *like* all of each other's friends, but you do have to respect each other's relationships.

If the man you're thinking of marrying does things that you don't like—say he goes out and gets drunk with his friends twice a week and you *hate* it —don't expect him to change after you're married. He may stop doing it (whatever it is) but only when and if *he* wants to. If you're going to marry someone, you have to like him the way he is, or at least be sure that you can live with the things that you don't like. You're going to be disappointed if you expect a man to change his ways just because you've married him.

The considerations about whom you marry and if you marry are the same no matter how old you are.

But the reason that young marriages so often fail is that younger people tend to be less careful about choosing their mates than older people, though older people certainly do make plenty of mistakes. Are you thinking of getting married simply to get away from your parents? Or because you're pregnant? Or because it's so much more difficult to have sex when you're not married? Are you considering only one factor in the decision to marry? There *are* other solutions to any of these problems. You have other ways of getting away from your family, other ways of coping with an unplanned pregnancy, and, if you think about it creatively, ways to make your sex life better without getting married. You and your boyfriend may be desperate to spend a whole night together, but marriage means that you'll be spending a lot of nights and a good part of your days together too.

The picture for a young marriage isn't entirely bleak. There have been good ones. But the good marriages, at whatever age, are made by people who each have a strong sense of who they are and what they want to do *individually,* and are building their relationship on their individual strengths. They're not depending on marriage to make them complete people or to solve their problems.

And then, finally, there's an element of luck involved. You'll both continue to grow after you're married. You may find that you're both growing in more or less the same direction, or you may find yourselves, after a few years, at odds in terms of values, goals, life-styles. Certainly being married doesn't mean that you have to do and think all the same things (which is impossible anyway, if you're being honest with yourself), but if you wind up disagreeing about the things that are most important to you, that means serious trouble for the marriage.

No relationship, even a marriage, is so important that it's worth compromising yourself for the sake of the relationship. It's nice to have someone to love, and it's nice to be loved. And it's nice to feel that you're the most important person in the world to someone else. But none of this will make you happy unless you like the person you are.

5

Sex

A hundred years ago, an unmarried woman was not supposed to know anything whatsoever about sex, and she was certainly not supposed to *do* anything about it if she did know. Sex was something she learned all about on her wedding night, if she had one, and she was never expected to enjoy it. Not everyone fitted exactly into that pattern, but at least a woman knew what was expected of her. This system had drawbacks for many women. Some found they enjoyed sex when they weren't supposed to, and many others never got to enjoy it at all. But most women then undoubtedly felt less confused about sex than many women do today.

Today we're faced with a situation that's much less clear. We're told there has been a sexual revolution, and that is supposed to mean that women are free to have and enjoy all the sexual relationships we want. The idea of the sexual revolution has partly replaced the belief that "nice" girls shouldn't have sex before marriage. Some people will tell you that it's okay to have intercourse if you're planning to get married *or* if you're really in love. Some people will argue that sexual experience before marriage is important to a good adjustment after marriage. And some people will tell you that sex should be as natural and uncomplicated as eating and sleeping and that you should just do it when you want to. And there are still many people who believe that teenagers shouldn't have sex at all. Meanwhile, you're still an individual and have to make decisions that are good for *you*. If anything, that's harder than it used to be, just because of all the conflicting things that you hear. There's no one answer that's right for everyone or even for most people. The important consideration is not what you do, but how you feel about it.

Sex isn't something that you suddenly become interested in when you reach adolescence. Tiny babies discover that touching their genitals (sex organs) is very pleasant, and most little children play doctor, looking at and feeling one another's genitals. Many parents, if they discover this, get upset and punish their children for it. Punishment, of course, won't stop their children's interest; instead, it forces them to do the same things secretly and gives them the idea that there's something wrong with what they're doing. Some parents do understand that there's nothing wrong with masturbation and sex play in young children, but even children with parents like these may get the idea from other children or adults that there's something wrong. So most of us grow up with the attitude that there's something peculiar about sex.

Some societies expect and permit sexual activity in people of all ages. Little children openly play sexual games and teenagers are expected to have sexual intercourse. While everyone in our society knows that most teenagers are interested in sex, the most common attitude is that you're not supposed to *do* anything about it. If everyone believed that sexual activity (which includes masturbating, kissing, necking, petting, intercourse, and all the possible variations) is normal and healthy for teenagers, it wouldn't be so hard for you to find a place to have sex, and the decisions *you* have to make about sex wouldn't be so complicated.

Some "experts" recently suggested that, since teenagers prefer to make out in their own homes, parents of teenagers should be sure that at least one parent is *always* home, so they always know what is going on. I suppose those experts would also recommend that the parents take turns sleeping, just to be on the safe side. They don't give teenagers enough credit, since if you want to do something enough, you'll certainly be able to find some place to do it. The decisions about sex are complicated enough, but they don't seem to be affected much by how closely your parents watch you.

Who Knows What's Right for You?

Parents generally tend to be stricter with girls than they are with boys, as you probably already know. If a mother discovers a rubber in her son's pocket, she'll probably be surprised and maybe amused. If your mother finds a package of birth control pills in your drawer, you're probably in for a bad scene, unless you have a pretty unusual relationship with your mother. If parents were able to be open about sex with their children, it would be possible to get help from them with your own decisions. But that's a rare situation, and even teenagers who have parents they can talk to sometimes don't want their parents to know everything that's going on. You have a right not to talk to your parents about things that don't affect them directly, if you don't want to.

Many of the popular books about sex, which many people look to for advice, like *The Sensuous Woman,* or *Everything You Always Wanted to Know about Sex but Were Afraid to Ask,* or *The Happy Hooker,* are full of misinformation and fantasy. What they tell you is that if you know the right tricks, sex won't be a problem for you. Just knowing what to do and how to do it, though, isn't going to help you *decide* what to do and when and with whom. What these books hint at is that if your sex life is good, then the rest of your life will be too, and that simply isn't true.

Whatever advice you get and whatever pressures

you face, you are the one who has to decide what to do about sex in any particular situation. In some schools or social groups, there are informal sets of "rules" about what is all right to do when. For instance, you can kiss on the first date, neck on the second, pet above the waist on the third, or whatever. Nobody pays much attention to rules like that, although everyone seems to say they do. Anyway, they don't solve your problem if you find that you want to pet on the second date or that you don't want to neck on the third.

These rules also raise some peculiar questions like: If a boy takes you out on Saturday, walks you home the next Wednesday, and then takes you out again on Friday, is Friday the second date or the third? Making rules about making out can also get terribly complicated. You can figure out (if you want to bother) a hundred gradations of above the waist, outside your clothes, bra on, bra off, below the waist, etc., etc. What none of the rules takes into account is what *you want* to do. Since you have a head attached to the body that all this is happening to, you'll have to use it to decide what you're going to do.

Since your body and your head are both parts of your self, the trick is to get them working together. Your body gives you signals all the time. Sometimes you pay attention to them; sometimes you don't. You can control your body's signals to some extent. If you're running a race and get tired, you can sometimes will yourself to stop feeling tired and go on. Especially where sexual feelings are concerned, you may find that you're getting different signals from your body and your mind.

Masturbation

Masturbation (which means touching or rubbing your genitals with your hand or something else for pleasure) is one way of getting to know your body sexually. It's the one kind of sexual activity that doesn't involve another person, which uncomplicates things somewhat, since you don't have to worry about what another person is doing or feeling or thinking. Young people used to be told that masturbating was wrong, that it could make you blind or crazy. More recently, it's been realized that masturbating is normal (that is, nearly everybody does it and likes it), but you may have heard that you shouldn't do it too much. Of course, no one tells you exactly what "too much" is. But your body can tell you: When your genitals get sore, you're masturbating too much. However, you'd have to be masturbating an awful lot for that to happen, so you probably don't have anything to worry about. The only other "too much" would be if you gave up most of your other activities in order to masturbate all the time. However, it would be just as unhealthy if you gave up everything else in order to do nothing but stamp collecting or eating or anything else as a single all-consuming preoccupation.

If you feel like you want to masturbate, then there's no reason why you shouldn't. It's a good way to learn about your body and how it responds sexually. Masturbating is a good way to relieve the tension that you may feel if you've been making out and then you get home and find that you can't sleep because you're so tense. In fact, masturbating is a way of relieving tension whether you've been making out or not.

Sex: The Physical Part

In strictly physical terms, there are four stages of sexual response. The first is *excitement,* or arousal. In the excitement stage, your muscles start to stiffen, there is an increased blood supply to the genitals, you start breathing heavily, and your heart beats faster. In men, the penis becomes larger and erect. In women, the clitoris, which is a very sensitive little button of flesh between the lips of the vagina, becomes erect, and a thick, clear fluid is produced in the vagina and usually seeps out. The fluid is there to lubricate the vagina so the penis can enter easily.

Sexual excitement can start in all sorts of ways, which vary from person to person and from time to time for any individual. What turns you on may not turn on someone else; and what turns you on one day may not turn you on the next. Pictures, books, dreams, daydreams, certain kinds of physical activity, touching yourself or being touched are some of the things that can turn people on. The excitement phase can be stopped by a variety of things, again depending on the individual and the circumstances: hearing a sudden noise, or worrying about someone coming in, or being tired, or purposely thinking about something else. For a lot of women, the best way to get turned off is to have someone say, "What's the matter with you? Why aren't you getting excited?"

The second stage is called *plateau*. The changes that started with excitement continue. The breathing and heart rate increase, the muscles become more tense. In women, the clitoris, which has become extremely sensitive, withdraws between the lips. In men, the erection becomes even larger. If regular stimulation of the right kind continues once the plateau stage is reached, orgasm will occur. If you don't have an orgasm at this point, it takes the body several hours to get back to its normal state of breathing, heart rate, and muscle tension.

Orgasm is difficult to describe. Poets and novelists have sometimes done a reasonably good job of explaining what it feels like, but their descriptions are mostly helpful for people who already know what they're talking about. Scientists describe orgasm as a series of rhythmic contractions which are felt mainly in the genitals. These contractions release all the tension that has been building up. An orgasm lasts for three to ten seconds, though it may seem to last longer. It feels *very good*. In men, at the point of orgasm, there is an *ejaculation* (or spurting) from the penis of a fluid called semen. This fluid carries the sperm that can make a woman pregnant. There is no ejaculation for women. The fluid that you sometimes feel coming from the vagina is simply for lubrication, and it's there whether or not you have an orgasm.

In a woman, the clitoris must be stimulated for her to have an orgasm. However, it doesn't have to be touched directly. Some women can stimulate themselves to orgasm just by rubbing their legs together, and a few can get an orgasm just by thinking about sex. During sexual intercourse, since the penis is in the vagina, it is not usually in direct contact with the clitoris. However, the lips of the vagina do rub against the clitoris, and for some women this stimulation is enough to bring them to orgasm. A lot of women, however, don't have orgasms unless the clitoris is stimulated more directly with a hand or a mouth or an object.

The fourth and last stage of sexual response is called *resolution*. This is the period of time it takes for your body to get back to its normal state. This can take four or five minutes if you've had an orgasm, and four or five hours if you've reached plateau and not had an orgasm. The time is the same for men and women.

What's Going On in His Head?

When you're having sexual activity (of any kind) with another person, it involves more than just what feels good physically. How you feel about the other person and how that person feels about you is important. If you're just starting to have sexual experiences, it's hard to know how to act because you're doing things you've never done before. And the feelings that arise can be very strong. It can be hard to feel comfortable with those feelings, especially since it's not always clear how the other person feels. Since teenagers (and most adults, too) often have trouble talking about their real feelings, you may find that you spend a lot of time trying to figure out how that other person really does feel. But your partner is probably just as confused and having just as much trouble sorting things out as you are. You'd do better to give your energy to figuring out your own feelings and trying to talk to your partner about them.

Boys, even if they're older than you, are often not much more experienced or sure of themselves than you are, even if they try to act like they are. Teenage boys are at least as nervous around girls as teenage girls are around boys. Take a look at a dance and you'll see all of them sticking together in a bunch for protection from you. They are under pressure to look and act cool and to "get" as much (sexually) as they can from girls. Many boys would probably be happier without that pressure, so they too could learn to be themselves and not always have to keep up a front. The pressure on you is the opposite: to resist his demands as much as possible, by whatever means you can. What that doesn't take into account is what you want or need or feel comfortable with.

It's hard in this society for anyone to express their sexual needs honestly. If you do talk about what you want, you may be considered fast, or your partner may tell you you're being too aggressive. If the boy does, and puts pressure on you, you may get turned off to him. So what should be free and open gets complicated because people can't talk openly about what they want and need, and sex can turn into a game where everyone loses touch with themselves.

Saying No

The best time to decide what you will and won't do about sex is *before* you're actually faced with the decision. Once you're in the situation, you can always change your mind. But if you're making out with someone and he's putting pressure on you, it's hard to think clearly. Having made a decision earlier at least gives you something to go on and helps you stay in control of things. There are a number of things to consider when you make a decision; some involve you only, some involve the boy and your feelings about him, some involve a number of other people. Start with yourself, since you're the one who's most important.

If there's something you don't like to do because it doesn't feel good to you, then don't do it. Sex should be pleasant for both of you, and there's absolutely

no reason to do it if it isn't. What any person likes
sexually varies. It's not only different for everyone,
but it changes from time to time for everyone. For
instance, some women like having their breasts
touched and some don't. You may find that you like
having your breasts touched most of the time, but
that just before your period they get very tender and
having someone touch them is annoying. At that
point, you can say no and explain why you're saying
no, if you want to explain.

You may know that you'll feel guilty if you do a
particular thing. That's another perfectly legitimate
reason for saying no. That's not to say that you
should feel guilty about sex. Guilt is a nasty and
rather useless emotion, one that should be avoided
as much as possible. But what you feel comfortable
doing is going to vary according to your age and
experience, the relationship you have with your
partner, your upbringing, and the attitudes of your
friends. If you *always* feel guilty about *any* sexual
activity, and if that doesn't change, you are going to
miss out on some nice experiences. The way to overcome guilt is by exploring the reasons for your guilt
and deciding if they make sense, not by repeating
the thing that made you feel guilty. If your reasons
do make sense, then you'll have to avoid doing whatever it was that made you feel guilty in the first
place. If your reasons for feeling guilty don't really
make sense to you—for example, if you *always* feel
guilty after any sexual activity, even when you've

enjoyed it—then admit to yourself that you have a problem. If you can't figure out the reasons for your guilty feelings by yourself, you might consider getting some counseling or therapy. Until you understand *why* you feel as you do, you'll have a hard time changing yourself.

Sex: Who With and What For?

Except for masturbation, sex involves another person, and how you feel about sex will be affected by who the person is and what the person does. Your body will tell you when you're physically ready for something. But just because you're sexually aroused, you don't *have* to have sex. Your feelings about the other person may not be right. The time or the place or something else may be wrong. The boy who turns you on may not be one you like or trust, though it's easy to be confused by that. We're taught that we're not supposed to have sexual desires for people we don't love. So sometimes when someone turns us on, we think it must be love, since that's what it's supposed to be. But if he wasn't lovable before, there's no reason for him to be lovable after. You might also find that you think you really like him when you're not with him, but when you see him, though you still get excited, you find all sorts of things wrong with him. What is happening is that you're creating a romantic picture of him that you can only manage to keep up when he's not there. And when you're faced with him in the flesh, the picture falls apart.

It's perfectly possible for you to like someone well enough to go out with but not enough to want to neck or pet. You have to assume that a boy asked you out because he wanted to be with you, not because he wanted to make out. You don't have to pay him with sex for the time and money he's spent. Some boys think, and will try to make you believe, that if they take you out someplace special (and expensive), you should be more willing than usual to make out. But you (and he) are still the same people, whether you've gone for a walk around the block or to a rock concert or to the senior prom.

It's possible to like a boy and still not trust him. In spite of the so-called sexual revolution, in most places it's still considered "all right" for boys to have a lot of sexual experience but not so all right for girls. Boys do talk about girls and about sex. (Girls also talk about boys and about sex, but that rarely does the same kind of damage.) There's usually no real way of knowing whether or not a boy will keep his mouth shut about what went on between you. However, if he tells you things about other girls he's gone out with, or if his friends have ever told you stories about him and girls he's dated, you can be sure you won't be the *one* girl he doesn't tell anyone about. Or you may just *feel*, without knowing anything specific, that he will probably talk. You should trust your own feelings in that case. If you continue seeing him for a while, without giving him much to tell his friends about, you may eventually get a clearer idea of whether or not you can really trust him.

Boys have also been known to make up stories about girls. Since boys are supposed to have a lot of sexual experience, they sometimes tell their friends about things that never really happened, and some of those stories could be about you. There's no easy defense against that. If you know (or suspect) that that's happening, you're probably wise to avoid the boy, and his friends too, for a while. Coping with a bad reputation isn't easy and needs all the dignity you can muster. Rather than try to deny the lies, try to ignore them. They're not worth your time. Your sex life is your own business, and if *you* are comfortable with it, you'll be better able to deal with whatever talk there may be.

Love and Sex

More women have probably been talked into having sex when they didn't want it by being told "I love you" than any other way. It may be we feel grateful for love, or that love represents so much of what we want (or are supposed to want) in life that we can't stand the thought of losing it. So if someone tells you he loves you, you really have to work to keep your wits about you. A lot of boys are aware of how well those three words work and deliberately use them to get girls to have sex. So he could be lying. Boys can also be genuinely confused about the difference between sexual desire and love, so he may not really be a nasty, lying person but simply a mixed-up one.

Maybe he does love you. Or maybe he believes he loves you (which is almost the same thing). What *you* do still depends on what *you* want. Being grateful, whether for love or for money spent, is no reason to have sex. If you feel you shouldn't have sex with someone you don't love (whether or not he loves you), then don't. Your feelings are as real as his, and there's no reason for you to ignore them. If he really loves you, your feelings will matter to him, and if you say no, he should be willing to respect your decision. Though he'll probably keep trying, and you can't blame him for that. His need for sex (like yours) may be perfectly real, and you can't expect it to go away. If he loves you, and you don't love him, you should be frank about the way you feel and give him the chance to break off a relationship which may be painful for him. That's only fair.

It's possible to love someone yet not want a sexual relationship. You can love someone but feel that you're still not ready to cope with sex. Or you may feel that you're just too young or that you're not sure enough of your feelings. Or you may believe that sex before marriage is wrong. Or you may not want to have to make a decision about birth control. Or you may just simply not want to, for no reason that you can explain. So don't. You don't have to have sex with someone because you love him. And don't let him tell you that you do. You don't have to feel that you must defend your right to say no, either. You don't have to give reasons and explanations, unless you want to. You don't have to prove your love with sex. If that's the only proof he'll accept, if he doesn't believe that you love him from the way you act toward him, then he's not going to believe you any more if you do have sex.

Sex doesn't necessarily go with love. You can have sex (of any variety) just because you feel like it, whether you love the person (or even like him) or not. Two people can be physically attracted, have great sex together, and have very little else in common. Once again, what you do in a situation should depend on what you want to do, what will make you happy, and not on someone else's ideas of what you should or shouldn't do. You are always the best judge of your own feelings.

Lines, Techniques, and Tactics

Boys and men are more open about expressing their sexual needs than are most women, and some of them will use their needs to pressure you into doing things you may not want to do. He may tell you that you are responsible for his erection and that you should therefore do something to relieve it. He may tell you that he's going to be permanently damaged if he doesn't have an orgasm immediately. He won't. If he gets very excited and doesn't have an orgasm, he'll probably be uncomfortable for a while, just as you would be. If you want to give each other the pleasure of an orgasm, that's fine. But if you don't, you don't have to let yourself be forced into it.

The boy may tell you that you led him on. It's a little tricky to figure out what is leading someone on and what isn't. What he's talking about is his response, and you may not have (or may not *think* you have) done very much to get him as turned on as he is. A lot of teenage boys do get very excited very easily. But unless you're purposely teasing him (and you *know* when you're doing that), you don't have to feel responsible for his sexual excitement, unless you want to. It can be just as hard for you to stop something as it is for him, and the burden shouldn't all fall on you. If you really enjoy necking (or whatever), then you should be able to do it without his telling you that you *must* go further.

The sex researchers, Masters and Johnson, have found some evidence that reaching plateau (the short stage just before orgasm) over and over again without ever having an orgasm can have bad effects. Sometimes a person gets so used to not having an orgasm that she (or he) is finally *unable* to have one. But this takes a long time to happen. Meanwhile, you (or he) can relieve any tension that you feel by masturbating or petting to orgasm. Since an orgasm, no matter how you get it, will relieve the tension, it isn't necessary to have intercourse unless you want to. About half of all women never have an orgasm during sexual intercourse anyway, but virtually every woman *can* have an orgasm if she's stimulated the right way. And the right way simply depends on what feels best to her. There's nothing good or bad about any method—anything that works for you and gives you pleasure is fine.

A boy may tell you that you're being a prude or a baby or old-fashioned or uptight if you don't do what he wants. The best you can do with that kind of accusation is try to ignore it. You have a right to do what you want to do. Having sex is not going to make you grown up or modern. Boys don't usually mean those things when they say them anyway. They're simply "lines" that sometimes get them what they want, so they may try them out. Don't let a boy tell you things like "You know you want it." You know what you want a lot better than he does.

Sometimes a boy threatens (straight out or by hinting) that if you don't do what he wants, he won't see you again. If that happens with someone you've just started going out with, there's not much you can do but write him off as being only interested in you for sex. If he starts right off by trying to get you to do things you don't want to do, the chances of a good relationship developing are slim anyhow. And there's no guarantee that he'll see you again even if you do what he wants.

That same kind of sexual pressure can arise in a good, ongoing relationship too, and then the problem is somewhat different. If you really like the boy and he likes you, then there's a desire to please each other. The idea that if he respects you he won't ask you to have sex doesn't take into account that his sexual feelings may be very real and very strong. Or it may be that you want sex and he doesn't, and again it's not fair to say that the feelings of the person who doesn't want sex are more important than the feelings of the person who does. Sometimes there's room for compromise. He may not want to have intercourse, but may still feel comfortable about petting to orgasm.

If you're in this kind of situation, try to think through your feelings by yourself and decide what you want and don't want and why. Then in a calm moment (not when things are already hot and heavy) you'll have to talk about the problem with him. If he likes you, he may be able to accept your feelings once you've explained them. If he refuses to discuss the situation or refuses to compromise, then you have to accept that there's something wrong with a relationship where your feelings aren't taken seriously. You can decide whether or not you want that kind of relationship. You can decide either way, but at least you'll know where you stand.

Sometimes, in spite of all your carefully thought-out decisions and your good intentions, you wind up getting "carried away" and doing something you wish you hadn't. That happens to almost everyone at one time or another. Since you can't undo what you've already done, the best thing you can do for yourself is not to let it make you miserable. Feeling guilty isn't going to help. You may find, after thinking about the experience, that it wasn't so bad after all. If you're still sorry about what you did, you may be able to be firmer about not doing it again.

If you're worried about your physical desires getting out of control, there are a couple of things you can try when you feel that starting to happen. You can force yourself to think about something else— like the homework you haven't done, or the fact that your clothes are getting messed up or that someone might come in and find you or that the boy might realize you're wearing a padded bra, or *anything* but what you're doing. Or you can brightly suggest getting something to eat (which *always* works with some boys). Or you can yell, "STOP!" which doesn't always work but is worth a try. What you have to do is somehow break the progress of what's going on.

Think First

Once you've decided that your feelings, physical and emotional, are right, and you've decided that you want to have sexual intercourse, there are a number of very practical decisions to be made. The main decision concerns birth control. *Hope* (that you won't get pregnant) *is not a method of birth control.* One out of every twenty girls gets pregnant the *first* time she has intercourse. And it *can* happen to you.

So it's something that you absolutely must think about. This is no time to get "carried away." You have to be responsible to yourself and protect yourself.

Your first experience with intercourse won't lose anything (and it might even be better) if you plan it a little. If you have the presence of mind to pick a time and place where you know you won't be interrupted, and if you don't have to worry about getting pregnant, it can only help. If you're going to have intercourse, then admit it to yourself, take it seriously, and be responsible for it.

First sexual intercourse, unless the boy is very experienced (and he probably isn't, even if he claims to be), is usually not great. In fact, if you've been petting to orgasm, you may find intercourse rather disappointing. You'll probably be nervous. The boy will probably be nervous. Two nervous people can't do anything terribly well, so don't be surprised if intercourse doesn't seem to be anything special at first. The boy, because of his excitement, may have an orgasm very quickly. The chances of your having an orgasm the first time are close to zero. You may be part of the 50 percent of women who don't usually have orgasms during intercourse. Or, if you're in the other 50 percent, you may find that you have to be very relaxed, and it will probably take some experience before that happens.

You should also be prepared to find that, because of his nervousness, the boy may not be able to get an erection. That happens to every male at some time or other, usually because he's nervous or tired or has something else on his mind. But your partner will probably feel embarrassed and generally terrible about it, especially if he can't get an erection the first time you two try to have intercourse. Don't tease him; don't laugh at him; don't put him down for it. He's not a different person from the one he was. And you can both be assured that the condition (which is called "impotence") isn't permanent, although the more worried he is, the more likely he is to be impotent the next time.

With regard to sex, as with anything else, the important thing is to try to be realistic about yourself and your needs and your feelings. It's a normal, healthy activity and can be an expression of love and joy, or an exciting and satisfying physical experience, or both. It can also be a way of letting yourself be used. For one girl, the decision to have intercourse at fifteen may be a perfectly correct one; another girl may not be ready until she's twenty-two or older. Whatever your age, what you do is up to you.

6

Anatomy, Menstruation, and Getting Pregnant
What They Didn't Tell You in Biology 101

If you have had a typical American education, you probably already know (or are supposed to know) more about pronouns and triangles and the Hundred Years' War than you do about your own body. When you do learn something about the human body, the information is usually crammed in at the end of a biology or hygiene course where you've spent the year learning everything you always wanted to know about amoebas and frogs. With rare exceptions, those schools that offer sex education give the course in the last year of high school, long after the information was first needed and after a lot of information (right and wrong) and attitudes (good and bad) have been picked up. You really need to know *everything* about your own body: how it's put together and how it works, what you have to do to keep yourself healthy and how to recognize when you're not— and you should start to learn all that in kindergarten. It's certainly more important to most people than the Hundred Years' War.

These next few chapters are not going to tell you everything you need to know about your body. But since your reproductive system is going through major changes at this time in your life, and since you're probably most curious about it, it's the most important part of your body to learn about now, along with learning about the differences between male and female development.

The changes that take place in your body during adolescence—growth of body hair, development of breasts, beginning of ovulation and menstruation, and changes in the sex organs that you can see—are all set off and controlled by chemicals called *hormones*. Hormones are chemicals produced in the body by small organs called *glands*. Everyone (male and female) has the same hormones, but each person produces them in different amounts and different strengths. Men generally have more of some and women of others. Differences in hormone production, as well as differences in nutrition and general health, are why some people start to show the changes of adolescence earlier than others. There's nothing good or bad about developing earlier or later, although being the first or the last of your group to develop breasts or get your first period may make you uncomfortable for a while. Try to remember, if you're the first, that everyone will catch up very soon; if you're the last, you're the one who'll soon be catching up. Either way, there's usually nothing to worry about. The age when the changes start is determined by heredity to a large extent, and there's nothing you can do about that. If you haven't started to develop and you're concerned about it, you can see a doctor, who will examine you to make sure that you're healthy and will treat you if you're not.

Breasts

One of the most obvious things that has happened or will happen to you is that your breasts start to get bigger. Most of the breast is fat; the rest is made up of glands that can produce milk, and *ducts* (tubes) that carry the milk to the *nipple*. As the breast gets larger, so do the nipple and the *aureola*, which is the dark area surrounding the nipple. You may develop some hair between the breasts or around the nipples. This too is normal. The milk glands and ducts are usually inactive until late in pregnancy. Although the breasts exist so that a woman can feed her baby, not every woman chooses to breast-feed. What's more important to many women is that their breasts are sensitive to stimulation and they can get pleasure from having their breasts stroked or nibbled or sucked.

Your breasts, once they reach their full growth, don't always stay the same size. They get larger during the two weeks before your period and may become quite tender during the few days just before your period. In some women, the change in breast size is noticeable (at least to the woman herself; others are hardly aware of it). Your breasts may also get larger if you take certain kinds of birth control pills, if you get pregnant, or if you breast-feed a baby. All these changes are temporary, however, and as soon as you stop taking the pill or stop being pregnant (by having a baby, a miscarriage, or an abortion) or stop breast-feeding, your breasts will return to their original size. It's also not uncommon for a woman to have one breast that is larger than the other.

Many women are unhappy with their breasts for one reason or another. They think their breasts are too small or too large or too low or not the right shape. If you have small breasts, it may surprise you to learn that girls with large breasts are often self-conscious, and vice versa. Don't worry if you don't look like the models in *Playboy*. In most of the pictures, you'll notice that the model has her arms up over her head. Undress and look at yourself in the mirror. Then raise your arms over your head. If you like the effect, you can walk around with your arms over your head all the time. Or you can decide that you like what you see. After all, it's you. You can exercise the muscles that surround the breasts by doing push-ups or isometrics. That won't make your breasts any larger, but it will strengthen the chest muscles so they'll hold your breasts up better.

The Outer Genitals

About the time that your breasts develop, you'll notice some other changes starting to take place. Among the more obvious changes, hair starts to grow on various parts of the body—under your arms and around your genitals—and the outer lips of the vagina start to become larger and fatter. Both the hair around the genitals and the fleshy lips (which are called the *vulva*) are there to protect the delicate tissues underneath.

If you spread the *outer lips* of the vagina while looking in a mirror, you'll see that there is a second, thinner pair of lips lying between the outer ones. These are called the *inner lips.* They are usually pink or reddish, except during pregnancy when they become more purple. Directly between the inner lips are two openings, and below (or behind) these is a third. The opening most toward your back is the *anus,* through which come your bowel movements. It's the end of your digestive tract and is not connected to your reproductive system. The middle opening (the next one up toward the front of your body from the anus) is the *vagina.* The vagina is where the penis goes during sexual intercourse, and it is the canal through which the menstrual blood flows and through which the baby comes during childbirth.

The opening of the vagina may be partially covered by a membrane (or layer of skin) called the *hymen* or maidenhead or "cherry." If you do have a hymen (not all women are born with one), it has a hole in the center. The hole is usually large enough to insert a finger or two into it. It's also large enough, as a rule, to put a tampon into. The hymen is often broken the first time a woman has sexual intercourse. The breaking of the hymen is sometimes uncomfortable or slightly painful, sometimes painless, but rarely very painful. There is sometimes a little bleeding when it breaks. The hymen can also be stretched or broken without intercourse. If there is enough of an opening in the hymen, you'll be able to see a little way up the vagina.

The third opening between the inner lips, the one closest to the front of your body, is the smallest and hardest to find (it lies just above the opening of the vagina). It is the opening of the *urethra,* through which you urinate. It is connected to the *bladder,* where urine is stored.

The inner lips meet above the urethra and extend around the *clitoris,* forming the *clitoral hood.* The clitoris is a small button of flesh, which you'll find, if you touch it, is very sensitive. It is full of nerve endings and is the most sensitive spot on the human body. The vagina, on the other hand, contains very

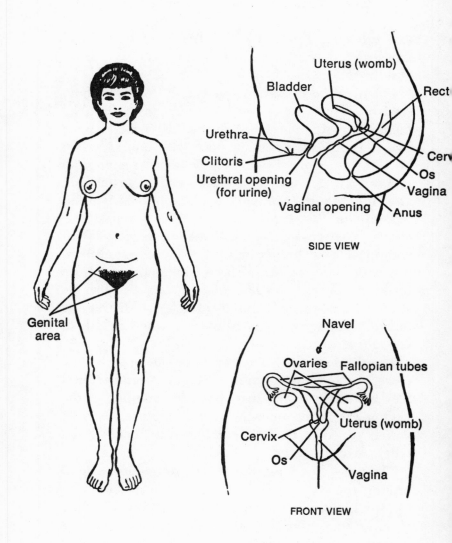

Uterus (womb)

Bladder

Rect

Urethra

Clitoris

Cer

Urethral opening
(for urine)

Os

Vaginal opening

Vagina

Anus

SIDE VIEW

Navel

Ovaries   Fallopian tubes

Cervix

Uterus (womb)

Os

Vagina

FRONT VIEW

Genital
area

few nerve endings. The pleasant sensations felt during masturbation or petting or intercourse are centered in the clitoris, even when it is not being touched directly. The only function of your clitoris is to respond to stimulation.

The Female Reproductive System

From its opening between the inner lips, the vagina extends three to four inches, aimed generally toward the small of the back. At the end of the vagina is a nipplelike projection with what feels like a dimple in the middle. You can feel it with a finger if you try. This projection is called the *cervix.* It is the extension of the uterus or womb into the vagina. The dimple in the center surrounds a very small opening to the uterus. This opening, called the *os,* is usually nearly closed and is too small for a tampon, for instance, to get into. But it can stretch to let bits of tissue pass through during menstruation or to allow a baby to pass through during childbirth. The vagina ends behind the cervix and has no opening at the back except for the os.

The *uterus* or womb is where the baby grows when a woman is pregnant. It is muscular, triangular (the cervix forms the lowest point of the triangle), and about the size of a tightly clenched fist. In a woman who is not pregnant, the uterus lies flattened between the *rectum* (the lowest part of the intestines) and the *bladder,* but it is not connected to

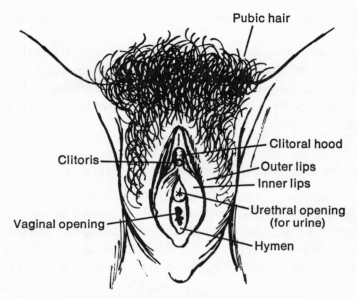

Pubic hair

Clitoral hood

Outer lips

Inner lips

Urethral opening
(for urine)

Hymen

Clitoris

Vaginal opening

DETAILED VIEW OF FEMALE GENITAL AREA

either one. The top of the uterus usually points forward toward the belly. If a doctor tells you that you have a tipped or retroverted uterus, it means that the top of the uterus points up or toward your back. This rarely causes any problems and is in fact quite common.

At either side of the top of the uterus, and opening into it, are the *Fallopian tubes*. If you can imagine that the upper part of your body is the uterus, your extended arms would represent the Fallopian tubes. Each is about four inches long. The ends of the Fallopian tubes (the points farthest from the uterus) are fringed. Each of the "fingers" of the fringe has a tiny opening. Lying just below the ends of the Fallopian tubes, but not directly connected to them, are the *ovaries*. Thus, there is one ovary on each side of the abdomen. Each ovary is one and one-half to two inches across and is oval in shape.

The Menstrual Cycle

Each ovary contains thousands of tiny, undeveloped eggs, which are already there at birth. In the course of your life, about three hundred of these eggs will mature. The eggs that do not mature remain in the ovary and are involved in producing hormones. Starting around the time that you get your first menstrual period, an egg matures and is released from an ovary approximately once a month. This process is called *ovulation*. It has very recently been discovered that most women ovulate every month from the same ovary (not one month from one ovary, the next month from the other, as most of us have been taught). The other ovary ovulates only occasionally, though it produces hormones. If the "active" ovary is removed, the "inactive" one will begin producing eggs. Most women who have only one ovary are as fertile as women who have two. Some women occasionally ovulate from both ovaries at once.

Your menstrual cycle is counted from the *first* day of one menstrual period to the first day of the next. The average menstrual cycle is usually considered to be twenty-eight days. However, the length of the cycle varies from woman to woman. Yours may be about nineteen days or about forty days or some other length. It takes a couple of years after you get your first period for your cycle to become regular.

The Ovarian Cycle

You are probably most aware of your menstrual cycle when you have your period, but important changes are going on during the rest of the month as well. Each month, at about the time your period starts, an egg starts to mature in one ovary and moves to the surface of the ovary. About two weeks later (on the average) the egg breaks through the surface and is released into the body cavity. Some women feel a little pain on one side of the abdomen when this happens. By a process which no one really understands, the egg is taken up into the fringed end of the Fallopian tube. This pickup process works extremely well. In women who have only one tube (because they were born with only one or have had one removed surgically), that tube can somehow attract an egg from the ovary on the other side of the body. The egg cannot move by itself, but is carried down the tube by movements of the tube and the tiny hairs called *cilia* which line it. It takes several days for the egg to get down the tube to the uterus.

Starting from the last day of your period, the lining of the uterus begins to grow and get thicker. This lining is prepared in order to protect and nourish the baby in a pregnant woman. If you do not get pregnant in any given month, about fourteen days after the release of the egg from the ovary, the lining of the uterus is cast off along with the egg and some amount of blood. All of this passes out through the vagina. The shedding of the uterine lining is your menstrual period. The blood and tissue passed usually amount to no more than a quarter of a cup, though it often looks like more. The "clots" you may notice are actually little pieces of the uterine lining.

In some societies, there's a big celebration when a girl starts to menstruate. We don't do that here, and too many girls in our society are still afraid or ashamed when they get their first period. It should be an occasion for rejoicing, though you may well have to rejoice alone. It means that you're growing up and your body is doing what it's supposed to do. If you don't menstruate by the time you're sixteen or seventeen, it's worth mentioning to a doctor. The age at which you start is determined mainly by heredity (the women in some families seem to start early, the women in other families start later) and partly by your general physical condition. Poor nutrition can delay the start of menstruation, as can a long illness or a number of other physical and emotional factors.

The Hormone Cycle

The whole menstrual cycle is controlled by hormones which also can affect the way you feel. Many women, though certainly not all women, feel rotten for a couple of days before their menstrual period. You may find that you are unhappy, short-tempered, and tired. You may have also noticed that your mother is periodically unhappy, short-tempered, and tired. It's not all in your mind. The emotional effects of the changing hormone levels in your body are absolutely real, and those changes can cause you or any other women to feel unhappy for a few days a month.

If you keep track of your cycle (that is, if you mark on a calendar the times when you get your period), you'll know if you're feeling awful because your period is due. Knowing that usually makes it easier to cope with—at least you know you're not going to feel that way forever. You'll probably also find that when you're feeling generally happy with your life, you won't notice the premenstrual (before your period) symptoms so much. Keeping busy helps, if you feel up to it, and some women find that getting more rest than usual makes them feel much better. While you have your period, you can swim, go horseback riding, have sex, or do anything else you usually do, if you feel like it.

Pain during your period isn't all in your mind either. Some women have no pain at all during menstruation; a few have such terrible cramps or backaches that they have to stay in bed for a day or two each month. Most of us fall somewhere between those extremes. If you have severe cramps (or mild ones), aspirin and heat (a heating pad or hot-water bottle) are often helpful. If the pain keeps you from your usual activities, then you should see a doctor. If he says he can't do anything for you, or if he tells you that it's all in your mind, see another doctor. Not much is known about *dysmenorrhea,* which is the medical term for painful menstruation, but a doctor should at least give you something to ease the pain. In general, your periods may become less painful as you get older. And some women find that once they have a baby or an abortion, their periods are no longer so painful.

You should bathe or shower daily while you have your period. You can use either sanitary pads or tampons to absorb the menstrual flow. Bacteria which cause odor and possibly infection can grow on the pads, so the tampons are most hygienic. Tampons and pads come in different sizes. The large ones are for a heavier flow, the smaller ones for a lighter flow. You can use different sizes as required. Tampons can be used even if your hymen is intact. Packages of tampons and pads contain instructions on how to use them.

If your period becomes irregular, when it has been regular for a while, or if it changes suddenly (for example, if it is a *much* heavier or lighter flow than usual for several months), you should see a doctor about it. There are some changes that take place without there being anything wrong, but you should check with a doctor to be sure. If you suddenly stop getting your period, either you're pregnant or something is wrong. In either case, you should see a doctor promptly.

Menopause

At some point in a woman's life, usually between the ages of forty-five and fifty, she gradually stops menstruating. This process, which may extend over several years, is called *menopause*. It is caused by a gradual change in hormone levels in the body. Just as the physical and emotional symptoms of menstruation vary from woman to woman, so do the symptoms of menopause. The only universal thing is that all women eventually stop menstruating.

Some of the more common symptoms of menopause (some women don't get any of these and almost no one gets them all) are: hot flushes (a sudden feeling of heat from the waist up that may last from a few seconds up to about half an hour), headaches, backaches, and fatigue. Some women also become irritable and depressed. Many of the symptoms, like those you may get before your period, have to do with lower levels of certain hormones in the body. If the physical symptoms are especially annoying, a doctor can prescribe *estrogen,* a hormone, which usually works well to relieve the physical discomfort. Recent evidence shows that taking estrogen over a long period of time may greatly increase a woman's chance of developing cancer of the uterus, so it's advisable to use estrogen only for a short time, if at all. Those women who shouldn't take birth control pills, because of high blood pressure, diabetes, or other health factors, shouldn't take estrogen for menopause symptoms.

Nervousness and depression at menopause sometimes hit hardest those women who believe that the only important thing they can do is have and raise babies. For these women, the menopause, since it means that they can no longer have babies, marks the end of their productive life. Women who have developed interests outside their homes seem, as a rule, to have an easier time during menopause, possibly because they are busy and are therefore less aware of the symptoms. Any woman who is having physical or emotional difficulties because of menopause should be urged to see a doctor and to find an occupation (paid or not) that will be interesting and rewarding. Our society unfortunately doesn't make it easy for middle-aged women to feel that they are valuable human beings, so it is often up to the individual woman to find something useful and fulfilling to do.

Male Anatomy

A man has two outside sexual parts, the *penis* and the *scrotum* (a sac which contains the *testes* and which hangs behind the penis). The penis and the scrotum are connected by a series of glands and tubes which lie inside the body.

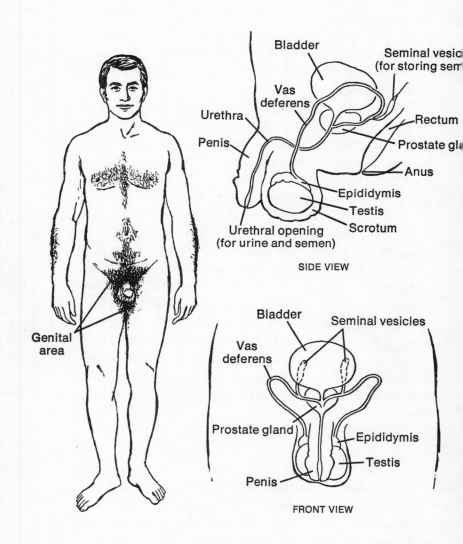

Genital area

Bladder

Vas deferens

Urethra

Penis

Urethral opening
(for urine and semen)

Seminal vesic
(for storing sem

Rectum

Prostate gl

Anus

Epididymis

Testis

Scrotum

SIDE VIEW

Bladder

Seminal vesicles

Vas deferens

Prostate gland

Epididymis

Testis

Penis

FRONT VIEW

The scrotum, which is very sensitive, contains two testes, which are a series of tiny tubes in which *sperm* are produced. Sperm are microscopic cells (that means you can't see them without a microscope). Each sperm has an oval head and a longer tail, which whips back and forth to move the sperm along. When a sperm from a man enters the egg in a woman's body, the egg is "fertilized" and a pregnancy will begin.

From the testes, the sperm move through a long (about eighteen-inch) tube, called the *vas deferens,* inside the man's body. From here, they are collected in the *seminal vesicles,* where they are joined by a lubricating fluid. When a man has an orgasm, the fluid, called *semen,* which contains the sperm, moves from the seminal vesicles past the *prostate gland,* into the urethra, and then out through the penis. This is called *ejaculation.*

The prostate gland, which contributes a little lubricating fluid, has another function. The tube from the bladder also passes into the prostate gland. The prostate controls whether urine or semen gets into the urethra and out the penis. The urethra in the man is a tube inside the penis which extends from the prostate to the tip of the penis. When a man is sexually excited, the prostate blocks the path from bladder to penis and the man cannot urinate until he is no longer aroused.

The penis itself is made up of spongy tissue. When a man is sexually excited, the penis becomes hard and erect. It does this because blood is being rushed to the blood vessels in the penis, and a muscle at the base of the penis, where it joins the body, contracts to keep the blood from flowing back out.

The penis, from the outside, has a smooth *shaft* and a *head,* which looks like a cap covering the end of the penis. Boys are born with a thin loose flap of skin, called the *foreskin,* covering the head of the penis. This is often removed by a doctor within a few days after birth, by a procedure called *circumcision.* If it has not been removed, the man must push the foreskin back daily and wash underneath it to remove a substance called *smegma* (a thick, cheese-like secretion) which collects there. If he doesn't do this, the smegma accumulates and may cause swelling and infection. (In a woman, smegma collects under and around the clitoral hood, so it is equally important that a woman wash this area regularly.)

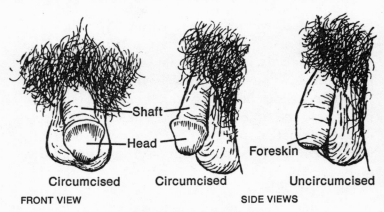

Circumcised   Circumcised   Uncircumcised
FRONT VIEW   SIDE VIEWS

PENIS AND SCROTUM

Conception and Pregnancy

When a man has an orgasm, 100 to 500 million sperm are ejaculated. If he ejaculates during intercourse, the sperm are deposited in the woman's vagina. The sperm can move by themselves, and unless something stops them, a certain number will swim through the cervix into the uterus and the Fallopian tubes. If there is an egg in the upper third of the Fallopian tube (the end near the ovary), it will be fertilized by a sperm, and the fertilized egg will be moved down the rest of the tube into the uterus, where it attaches itself to the uterine wall. At the time when the fertilized egg implants in the lining of the uterus and starts to grow, the woman is considered to be pregnant. It takes about a week from the time the egg is fertilized until it implants in the uterus.

Usually a woman ovulates (releases an egg from the ovary and into the Fallopian tube) about fourteen days *before* her *next* menstrual period. The egg can only be fertilized during the few hours (the exact time isn't definitely known) after it is released from the ovary. After that, the egg is apparently too "old." However, the "safe" period, or the time when you can't get pregnant, is difficult to figure out, especially for young women. Many women have irregular menstrual cycles, which makes it impossible to know definitely when your next period is due. Some women usually ovulate earlier or later in the cycle than the average. Usually a woman is fertile at some time in between her periods, but there are reported cases of women becoming pregnant while they were menstruating, although that's very unusual. Sperm can survive in a woman's body for up to a week, though most of them last only three to four days. The (relatively) long life of the sperm means that an egg can be fertilized by sperm that were ejaculated several days earlier, when the woman was supposedly "safe." (For more about calculating the "safe" period, see the section on the rhythm method of birth control in the next chapter.)

Once the fertilized egg is implanted in the uterine wall and starts to grow, a number of changes take place in the woman's body. The first thing that most women notice is that their periods stop. Since there are many reasons why a menstrual period can be delayed, it is always necessary to have a pregnancy test to confirm that pregnancy is the cause of the missed period. Other early signs of pregnancy *may* include tiredness, nausea and vomiting (since this often occurs in the morning, it is called "morning sickness"), frequent urination, and backache, though none of these alone is a reliable sign of pregnancy. Many women have no signs at all except the missed period, and a few women continue to have a light period for the first few months of a pregnancy. All of the signs of pregnancy are the result of changes in the hormones.

A pregnancy test can be taken about ten days after the missed period was due. That is, if your last period started on February 1 and you usually have a twenty-eight-day cycle, your period would have been due about March 1. If you didn't get your period by March 11 you could (and should) have a pregnancy test. Pregnancy tests are available from doctors, clinics, Planned Parenthood centers, free clinics, university health services, and sometimes from women's groups and hot lines. The woman's urine is tested; the test that most doctors and clinics now use takes about two minutes. The tests are not always absolutely accurate (though they're pretty good), so if the test is negative (meaning you're not pregnant), and if you still don't get your period, you should have another test in two weeks. If the test is still negative and if you still haven't got your period, you may need to have a more sensitive test done—or there may be some other problem. In either case, you'll need to see a doctor.

Pregnancy is calculated from the first day of the last menstrual period and, if it is not ended by miscarriage or abortion, usually lasts about forty weeks (or nine months). Thus, using the same example as before, if your last period started February 1, and if the pregnancy test was positive, you would be considered six weeks pregnant on March 15, and the baby would be due about November 7. The reason that pregnancy is calculated from menstrual dates rather than from the date of conception (when the egg was fertilized, which in this case would be about February 15) is that it's easier to know when your last period was than it is to figure out exactly when you ovulated.

Gynecological Exam

Gynecology is the branch of medicine that deals specifically with women, and a gynecological (or GYN) examination is an examination of a woman's genitals, reproductive system, and breasts. If you have a menstrual problem or a vaginal infection, if you need birth control, if you think you're pregnant, or if you suspect you have a venereal disease, you'll need to be examined by a doctor. Some family doctors and clinics will do a routine yearly GYN exam on any girl who has begun to menstruate. Other doctors will wait to do the first exam until there's a problem or until a girl requests it. A GYN exam can be done by your family doctor or by a specialist, called a gynecologist. Most gynecologists also practice obstetrics (which means that they deliver babies). I'm going to refer to doctors as "he" in this discussion, since in the United States, 93 percent of all doctors and 97 percent of all gynecologists *are* men.

A good GYN exam should begin with the doctor or an assistant taking your general medical history, as well as your family medical history and your own gynecological history. If you are seeing your family doctor, he probably has your medical history and your family history. Your GYN history includes:

What was the date (approximate) of your

first period? Is your period regular?
How long is your cycle (from one period to
the next) and is it changing?
How many days does your period last?
Is your period heavy, medium, light?
Do you have cramps or other discomfort
with your period?
Have you ever been pregnant?
How did the pregnancies end (childbirth,
miscarriage, abortion)?
What birth control method, if any, do you
use?
Do you have or have you had any infec-
tions or diseases or other problems?

Before you go to the doctor, write down the answers to these questions, as well as any questions
that you want to ask the doctor or any problems you
want to discuss. If you're seeing the doctor or going
to the clinic for the first time, write down the major
facts of your medical history: what diseases, conditions, or operations you've had and the dates, as well
as any allergies you have. Your family medical history includes whether anyone in your family (parents,
brothers, sisters, grandparents, and other blood rela-
tives) has had diabetes, tuberculosis, heart or circu-
latory disease, or cancer. If anyone in your family
has died, the doctor will want to know the cause of
death.

You have the right to have a nurse or another
woman in the room with you while you're being

examined. The doctor or assistant will tell you to undress and put on a gown, which they will provide. You can keep your shoes on or take them off, depending on how you're most comfortable. You're then weighed and your blood pressure is taken. The doctor may listen to your heart and lungs and look at your throat, ears, and eyes. If all this has been done in another part of the clinic or recently by another doctor, it isn't necessary to have it repeated. But since so many of us only see doctors when we have

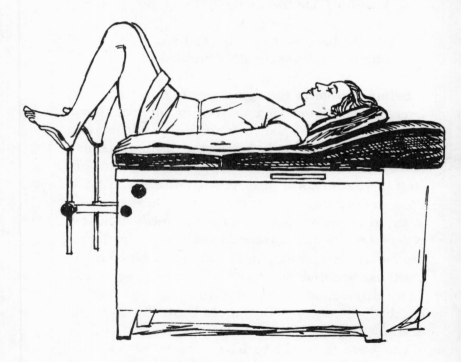

PATIENT IN POSITION FOR GYN EXAM

to, you can ask the gynecologist to do a general examination if you haven't had one in a while.

For the GYN exam itself, you'll be asked to lie on your back on an examining table, with your feet in special supports called stirrups. The doctor should then examine your breasts, thoroughly and gently. He may start the breast exam while you're sitting up. Once you're lying down, he'll ask you to put your hands behind your head. Then he will gently feel the entire breast, a little at a time, probing all the way into the armpit, to determine if there are lumps. Ask him to teach you how to do a breast exam yourself (he may give you a booklet which explains it), and you should then do a breast exam on yourself every month right after your period ends. Before and during your period, your breasts may normally be tender and lumpy, which makes it hard to tell if there are any abnormal lumps. (If you ever find a lump, let the doctor know about it immediately. It's probably a cyst, which is nothing to worry about, but any lump should be checked by a professional.)

After the breast exam (or before), the doctor will press and poke your abdomen from the outside. He'll be able to tell you if your organs are normal or enlarged. Tell him if you feel pain when he presses a particular spot.

He'll then examine your outer genitals for signs of infection or growths. Then he inserts two gloved fingers into the vagina. He'll find the cervix and hold it steady with his fingers so that the uterus can't move around. He then presses on the lower abdomen from the outside with the other hand. By doing this he can tell if there are growths on the uterus, or if you're pregnant, or if everything is normal. He'll feel for the Fallopian tubes and ovaries, which he probably won't be able to locate exactly unless they are enlarged for some reason. You may be able to tell when he locates an ovary, since you may feel a twinge of pain. This is normal. If the ovary is enlarged because of cysts or infection, he'll be able to find it easily. Some women periodically develop ovarian cysts, fluid-filled sacs that can grow to the size of an orange and disappear again by themselves in the course of one or two menstrual cycles. So they're usually nothing to worry about. Occasionally, when cysts grow very large and don't go away, they have to be removed surgically.

The next step in the GYN exam is internal examination with a speculum. Most doctors don't perform speculum examinations on women who have unbroken hymens unless there's a suspected infection or an indication of some other problem. The speculum is an instrument that holds the walls of the vagina open, so that the doctor can see the vaginal walls and the cervix. If you want to see all this for yourself, you can ask the doctor to hold a mirror at the opening of the vagina, so that you can see what he is seeing. He checks the color of the walls and the cervix and looks for discharges, growths, or damage. (It is important not to douche before you go to have a GYN exam so that any secretions are not washed away.)

While the speculum is in place, the doctor will

take a cotton swab and gently remove a few cells from the cervix. He then smears these on a glass slide and sends the slide to a laboratory, where a Pap test is done. A Pap test is a test for cancer of the cervix. You should have one once every two years until you're thirty; then yearly or oftener for the rest of your life.

The doctor should also take some fluid from the cervix and the urethra to be tested for gonorrhea. Some doctors order a gonorrhea test routinely for all their patients. With many doctors, however, you have to ask to have the test done. It can be embarrassing to ask a doctor to do a gonorrhea test, but because so many women who have gonorrhea have no symptoms, and because it's a widespread and serious disease, you should try to overcome your embarrassment and get a test regularly. The doctor should also draw some blood from a vein in your arm for a syphilis test. He may also have other blood tests done.

The most important thing you can do while your examination is going on is try to stay as relaxed as possible. If you get tense, the exam is uncomfortable because the muscles around the opening of the vagina tighten and the doctor has to force the speculum or fingers in. The more you can relax, the less discomfort you'll feel and the quicker the exam will be over. Consciously try to relax yourself, take deep breaths, think about something else. The GYN exam only takes a few minutes.

Once the exam is over, you get dressed and then

the doctor should see you to discuss any abnormal conditions he's found, answer your questions, and write any prescriptions you need. If he prescribes medication or birth control, he should tell you what he's prescribing and what it's for, how much to take and how often, possible side effects, and things to avoid while you're on the medication. If he doesn't tell you everything you need to know, keep asking. If you haven't had a chance before this point in your visit to ask the questions you came in with, this is the time to ask them. Sometimes doctors seem to be in too much of a hurry to answer our questions fully and in language that we can understand. If you don't understand something, or if there's something you feel you can't ask the doctor, try asking the nurse. She may be more willing to spend a little time talking to you. If you get home and realize that there's something you forgot to ask or you realize that you still don't understand something, call the doctor or clinic and get it straightened out. You have a right to good medical care, and good medical care includes explanations you can understand about what's happening to your body.

7

Birth Control
What They Didn't Tell You in Biology 101

Once you've decided to have intercourse with someone, you have a responsibility to each other to prevent pregnancy when you don't want a child. A knowledge of the consequences of an unplanned pregnancy and the decision to protect yourself from an unwanted pregnancy *must* be a part of the decision to have intercourse. Since you will undoubtedly be in more trouble than the boy if you get pregnant, the decision about birth control is one that concerns you most, though you may want to discuss it with him since he must also be responsible. Too many boys just assume (or hope) that the girl is doing something about birth control and don't bother to think about it themselves. However, a boy should recognize his responsibility and be willing to share the problems and decisions with you.

The decision to practice birth control often seems to demand more maturity than the decision to have intercourse. With any kind of sexual activity there's always a temptation just to let it happen. Then you can always tell yourself that you didn't mean to do whatever you did but just got carried away. It would be perfectly all right to get carried away if the price of unprotected intercourse were not so enormous. If you have intercourse regularly for a year without practicing birth control, you have an 80 percent chance of being pregnant by the end of the year. Making a decision about birth control means that you are taking yourself and what you're doing seriously and that you plan to continue being responsible.

Birth control doesn't just happen. With most methods, you have to *do* something each time. And that means that you have to admit to yourself that you *may* have intercourse. Remembering to take your pill on schedule or putting on your diaphragm before a date doesn't by itself mean that you *have* to have intercourse. But you will be prepared if you do. Always remember that the final decision is still yours, whether you are wearing the diaphragm or taking the pill or not.

Even if you are depending on the boy to use a condom, unless you know for a fact that he'll have one with him, you'd be wise to carry some of your own. It may be very, very difficult for you to go into a drugstore and ask for condoms or to present a boy with one at the critical moment, but it still may be easier for you than dealing with being pregnant. The alternative is to postpone intercourse until he or you can get something. NEVER let a boy talk you into taking a chance "just this once." The risk is simply not worth it.

Once you've decided that you're going to have intercourse and you're going to protect yourself, you have to choose a method. There are a number of birth control methods that are quite effective. Most of them control fertility from the woman's end of things, rather than the man's. While this places most of the responsibility on you, it also lets you keep some sort of control on your own fertility. Since you are the one who's going to get pregnant, it's probably best that you are most in control, since at least some boys aren't terribly trustworthy.

Unhappily, there is no completely effective, absolutely safe, perfectly simple method of birth control except complete abstinence, which means not having intercourse at all. If you decide on abstinence as a method, you definitely will not get pregnant, as long as you always hold yourself to it. Aside from abstinence, however, there are, in general, two ways of preventing conception from taking place. The first is to put some sort of physical or chemical barrier between the man's sperm and the woman's ovum (egg), so that fertilization cannot take place. The second is to interrupt the woman's hormone cycle so that no egg is produced or so that the fertilized egg cannot survive in the uterus.

When choosing a method of birth control, you

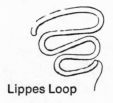
Lippes Loop

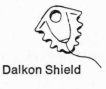
Dalkon Shield

IUD'S

Applicator for contraceptive jelly

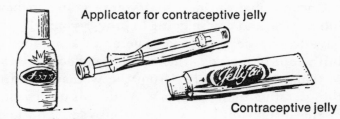

Contraceptive jelly

Contraceptive foam

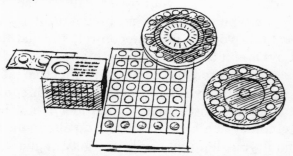

Varieties of birth control pills in different types of dispensers

CONDOMS

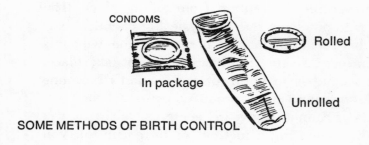

Rolled

In package

Unrolled

SOME METHODS OF BIRTH CONTROL

have to weigh the advantages and drawbacks in terms of your own life. You have to consider how often you have sex, your medical history, and how responsible you'll be about using a particular method. Most women use different methods at different times in their lives, as their needs and circumstances change. You can always switch from one method to another, if you're not happy with your choice. But don't just stop one method and then wait three months before you get another. That's a terrific way to get pregnant!

The Condom

The oldest and most widely used mechanical birth control method is the condom (rubber, safe, Trojan, Sheik, etc.). This is a thin rubber sheath that is fitted over the penis just before intercourse, after the penis is erect. When the semen is ejaculated, it stays inside the condom. Condoms are very effective *when used correctly.* First, they must be put on before the penis ever enters the vagina. When a man is sexually aroused, a few drops of lubricating fluid seep from the penis, and this fluid may contain enough sperm to make you pregnant. Second, the condom must be put on so that there is some room left at the tip for the semen. Otherwise, the condom may burst or the semen may leak out the back. Third, the penis must be withdrawn from the vagina soon after intercourse. Once the penis starts getting small again, there is danger that the condom will slip off inside the vagina and the semen will spill out. So soon after the boy ejaculates, he should hold the condom firmly around the penis at the end near his body and pull it out slowly. Brand name condoms, incidentally, are all checked before they are packed and do not have holes in them. You should avoid the kind that are sold in vending machines, since they are less reliable. Saran Wrap is no substitute for a condom, since there is no way to get it to fit well enough around the penis to keep the sperm inside.

Condoms can be bought in any drugstore. The usual price is about three for one dollar. They are generally used only once, though it is possible to wash, powder, and reroll them to use again. Some of them are made extra thin, so as not to cut down on the feeling that the man gets from intercourse. Besides the fact that they are effective and easy to get, condoms have another advantage over most other birth control methods: they give very good protection from venereal disease for both of you.

The Diaphragm

The diaphragm is another mechanical method of birth control. It is a soft rubber dome which is fitted over the cervix inside the vagina. The diaphragm *by itself* doesn't offer much protection, so it is always used with a sperm-killing cream or jelly. The jelly (or cream) is what actually protects you, but since the diaphragm holds the jelly in place so that the sperm can't get by it, the combination is *much* more effective than the jelly alone.

The diaphragm must be fitted by a doctor, who should also teach the woman how to put it in and take it out. MAKE SURE that the doctor has you practice putting it in, so that you know when it's on properly. Some doctors will try to rush you out before you're sure of what you're doing. If a diaphragm isn't positioned correctly, it may not work.

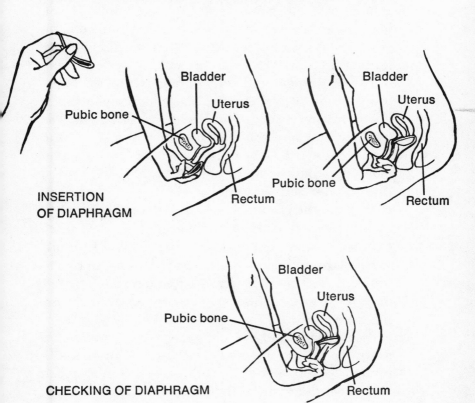

INSERTION
OF DIAPHRAGM

Bladder
Uterus
Pubic bone
Rectum

Bladder
Uterus
Pubic bone
Rectum

CHECKING OF DIAPHRAGM

Bladder
Uterus
Pubic bone
Rectum

No longer than two hours before intercourse, it is covered with jelly, folded, and pushed up into the vagina, just behind the pubic bone. Then you reach up and make sure that it is covering the cervix completely. The diaphragm is held firmly in place by the pubic bone and the walls of the vagina. After intercourse, it is left in place for eight hours to make sure that all the sperm in the vagina are dead. Then you pull it out, wash it, dry it, sprinkle it with cornstarch, and put it away until the next time. If you have intercourse again before the eight hours are up, you should insert more jelly with a special applicator that comes with the diaphragm.

The diaphragm with jelly or cream is a very effective method of birth control, as long as you use it *every time* and use it right. It's not as complicated as it may sound, and you'll get used to it quickly. If you have it fitted before or shortly after the first time you have intercourse, the fit should be checked by the doctor after a few months, since your size may change slightly. It should also be checked after childbirth or abortion or if you gain or lose more than ten pounds. Diaphragms range in size from fifty to one hundred millimeters, which is about two to four inches. A properly fitted diaphragm can't be felt once it's in place, either by you or your partner during intercourse.

Ramses jelly and Delfen cream are most effective as sperm-killing agents to be used with the diaphragm. Even though both are advertised for use without a diaphragm, they are much less effective when used alone (see next section). Koromex cream and Koromex jelly, both made to be used with a diaphragm, contain mercury and should be avoided, especially if you have kidney problems. The jelly or cream used with the diaphragm gives some protection from gonorrhea and other vaginal infections. But if you're going to use a diaphragm, you *must* use it every time, whether you think you're "safe" or not —and that includes using it if you have sex while you have your period. It can't protect you from pregnancy when it's home in your drawer.

Many doctors and birth control counselors don't tell teenage women about the diaphragm, because they don't believe that you can be consistent about using it. Only you can judge that, and if you feel that you're ready for it, and if you feel comfortable about touching your own genitals, *you* may have to tell that to the doctor and then be prepared to have him try to talk you out of it. Because it has no side effects and doesn't interfere in any way with your body's functioning, it is actually a very good method for many teenagers.

Jellies, Creams, and Foams

There are sperm-killing preparations which are designed to be used without a diaphragm. These come in several forms: foams, jellies, creams, and suppositories. The foam is the most effective. All are inserted with a special applicator directly into the vagina shortly before intercourse. They are all available in drugstores without a prescription, and all are relatively inexpensive.

Contraceptive foam comes in an aerosol can with an applicator. Delfen and Emko are about the best known and are equally effective. Within a half hour before intercourse (*no more!*), an applicator full of foam is inserted deep into the vagina. The application must be repeated before each intercourse, and it's also a good idea to insert another dose after intercourse, unless you plan to lie flat on your back for several hours. The jellies and creams are used exactly the same way, but are *much* less safe. The foams spread out evenly inside the vagina, and therefore the sperm-killing agent has the best chance of blocking the sperm. They also tend to be least messy after intercourse, since they don't melt and run out as the jellies sometimes do.

Contraceptive suppositories, which are large tablets that are inserted into the vagina, are much less effective than foams or creams or jellies, because they don't always melt completely or evenly. They should be avoided. Under no circumstances should you try to use "feminine hygiene" suppositories (like Norforms) as a birth control method. They are not designed as contraceptives and they don't work.

Foam and Condom

The "combination method" of using foam and condom at the same time has a number of advantages. Both foams and condoms are available at drugstores without a prescription. Together they give almost perfect protection against pregnancy. Together they give almost perfect protection from venereal disease. And since both you and your partner are using something, neither of you has to be the only one responsible for birth control.

Intrauterine Devices (IUDS)

Intrauterine (which means inside the uterus) devices—loops, coils, rings, and shields—also prevent conception. No one is quite sure how they work, although there are several theories. They are small plastic or plastic and metal forms of various shapes which are inserted by the doctor into the uterus itself. Unless there are complications, the device (or

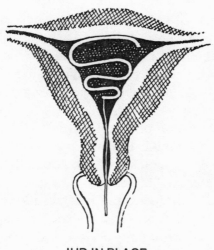

IUD IN PLACE

IUD) is left in until you want to get pregnant, when the doctor removes it.

The IUD is usually inserted while you have your period, since the cervix is soft and slightly open at this time. A narrow plastic tube, with the IUD inside it, is inserted through the cervix into the uterus. Then the IUD is pushed out with a plungerlike device (like a Tampax inserter, only smaller), the IUD is left in, and the inserter is withdrawn. This process may be uncomfortable, especially if you're tense about it or if the doctor isn't extremely careful and gentle. If you *are* nervous about the insertion, ask the doctor if he will use a local anesthetic. This is like the Novocaine the dentist uses.

There are two short nylon threads attached to the IUD. These hang down through the cervix into the vagina. If you have an IUD, you have to check to make sure that it's still there every week by reaching into the vagina and feeling for the strings. If you don't find them, it may be that the IUD has come out or is otherwise out of place, so you must use another method of birth control until you can get back to the doctor.

There are several problems with the IUD, especially for young women. If you have never been pregnant, there is a chance that the IUD will be pushed out of the uterus. This can also happen to a woman who *has* been pregnant, but it is less likely. You may not notice the IUD when it comes out, especially if this happens during your period, and you can be left unprotected. Another drawback to the IUD is that many women have unusually heavy menstrual bleeding and cramps for the first few months after insertion of the IUD. Sometimes these get so bad that the device has to be removed. Some women have bleeding between their periods, or they get a heavy white discharge from the vagina. The discharge isn't dangerous but can be annoying. Any unusual bleeding or discharge must be checked out with a doctor.

There is recent evidence that women who have IUDs may develop severe bacterial infections in the Fallopian tubes and ovaries. The infection is treated first with antibiotics; if the antibiotics don't work, one or both tubes and ovaries have to be removed surgically. Removal of one tube and ovary won't seriously affect a woman's ability to get pregnant. Removal of both ovaries not only leaves a woman sterile, but makes it essential that she take hormones to replace those normally produced by the ovaries. You should report to your doctor *immediately* any unusual discharge or any abdominal pain other than menstrual cramps.

IUDs come in various shapes and sizes. The smaller ones are retained best by women who haven't been pregnant. Unhappily, the smaller IUDs give the least protection from pregnancy. They are by no means a perfect method of birth control, and many women get pregnant with the IUD still in place. Sometimes the IUD causes an early miscarriage, but often the pregnancy continues for the full nine months. If it does, there is no risk to the baby from the IUD, which most doctors will leave in place if a woman becomes pregnant. There is usually less risk from an IUD which is left in place than from possible damage if it's taken out.

Some of the IUDs, in particular the Dalkon Shield, seem to make a woman more likely to develop an infection in the uterus around the middle of the pregnancy. An intrauterine infection is always fatal to the baby, and occasionally fatal to the mother. For this reason, most Planned Parenthood clinics have stopped using the Dalkon Shield. Planned Parenthood has recommended that women who have Dalkon Shields in place have them removed and replaced with another device or begin using another method entirely. Many doctors and clinics are calling in patients who have Dalkon Shields to advise them of the potential problems and to offer alternatives.

Occasionally (about once in twenty-five hundred insertions) the IUD gets pushed through the wall of the uterus and into the abdominal cavity (where your intestines are). If the IUD is one of the "open" kind, in which the ends of the device are not joined (Lippes Loop, Dalkon Shield or Saf-T-Coil), and if it goes all the way through the uterine wall, it is often left where it is and usually causes no trouble. If, however, the device which perforates is a "closed" model (Birnberg Bow or Hall-Stone Ring, in which the ends meet to form an 0 or an 8), there's a possibility that a loop of the intestine will fall through it and get caught. This is extremely serious, and the device has to be removed by surgery. Because of the seriousness of this complication, the closed devices should *never* be used. If you are going to get an IUD, try to find a doctor who has inserted a lot of them. He'll be most likely to insert it correctly, with the minimum possible discomfort for you.

An IUD called the Majzlin Spring has been withdrawn from the market by the Food and Drug Administration because it is very difficult to remove even when properly in place. In some cases, surgery has been necessary to get the Majzlin Spring out of the uterus. Don't let anyone insert a Majzlin Spring, Hall-Stone Ring, or Birnberg Bow. They've all been taken off the market because they can be dangerous, but some doctors and clinics have large supplies on hand and are continuing to use them. Ask what kind of IUD you're getting, and if it's one of these, insist on another kind.

Since no one knows just how the IUD works, no one knows exactly why it fails. But since it's only 80 to 90 percent effective in preventing pregnancy, and since there are so many potential problems, you may want to choose a less drastic method of birth control, at least for now. The advantage of an IUD is that, once it's in place, you only have to check it weekly, and you don't need to worry about it at all the rest of the time.

The Pill

The one widely used method of birth control that interrupts the ovarian cycle is the birth control pill.

Basically, what the pill does is change the normal cycle of hormone production so that there is no egg produced. It does this by putting artificial hormones into the body, which knock out the body's normal hormone production. The hormones in the pill prevent the body from producing the hormone that causes the release of the egg from the ovary. Since there is no egg to be fertilized, there can be no pregnancy.

There are two types of pills, the combination type and the sequential type. The combination type gives a small dose of *estrogen* and *progesterone* (two hormones) together for twenty or twenty-one days. The sequential type gives a dose of estrogen alone for fourteen or fifteen days, then progesterone alone for five or six days. Although the sequential pill copies the actual body cycle most closely, the dose of estrogen in these pills is higher than most women need to prevent pregnancy, so they are usually not recommended unless you have an estrogen deficiency (that means not enough estrogen in your body) to begin with. The sequentials are also slightly less effective in preventing pregnancy.

Birth control pills should be taken only on a doctor's prescription. Taking pills that were prescribed for someone else can cause you a lot of physical trouble. There are a number of conditions that the doctor will want to know about before he prescribes pills for you. The pills can be extremely dangerous to take if you already have liver or kidney disease, diabetes, migraine headaches, high blood pressure,

or a history of blood clots or breast cysts. The doctor
will also want to know if anyone in your family has
had high blood pressure, blood clots, diabetes, or
cancer. Once he knows your history, he can decide
whether or not it's safe for you to take birth control
pills, and he can warn you of things to watch for that
might be serious.

Some of the common side effects of the pill
("nonserious" because they won't kill you) are nausea, breast tenderness, weight gain, fluid retention,
mental depression, lower sexual desire, and increased risk of infection in the vagina. Any of these
should be reported to the doctor. In some cases, a
different pill will improve or correct the condition;
in other cases, you have to stop taking the pill before
the condition will clear up. Birth control pills give
no protection from venereal disease, and there is
some evidence that women who take pills are more
likely to get gonorrhea when they're exposed to it
than women who use other methods. The pills seem
to change the secretions in the vagina and make it
easier for germs to grow there.

Birth control pills are almost 100 percent effective
in preventing pregnancy, as long as you remember
to take them on schedule. Most pills are taken for
twenty or twenty-one days. Then you stop and you
get your period. Five days after your period starts
(counting the first day of your period as "day one"),
you start taking the pills again, whether you are still
bleeding or not. If you forget to take a pill, then take
two the next day, and use some other method of

birth control for the rest of that cycle while you continue to take the rest of the pills on schedule.

The long-term effects of the birth control pill are not yet known. Most doctors recommend that you have a checkup once a year when you're on the pill, and some doctors will want to see you every six months. Most doctors also recommend that you stop taking it for a few months every year or two to give your body a rest. Some doctors will not give the pill to young women, because they don't really know what effect it will have in the long run. It does interfere with your body's normal functioning, and you or your doctor may decide that the risk of permanently messing up your system just isn't worth it. A significant number of women have trouble getting pregnant when they stop taking the pill, and you may feel that you don't want to take that risk. The most serious side effect of the pill is the chance of getting blood clots in the lungs. Stop taking the pills and call your doctor *immediately* if you get chest pains, leg cramps, severe sudden headaches, blurring of vision, or if you start coughing up blood.

The Mini-Pill and the Morning-After Pill

There are a number of hormonal contraceptives being tested which may eventually prove to be safer than the birth control pills now on the market. One of these is the "mini-pill." This is a small dose of progesterone which is taken every day. Since most of the unpleasant side effects of birth control pills are caused by the estrogen in the pill, the mini-pill, because it contains no estrogen, eliminates most of the side effects. It prevents pregnancy, not by stopping ovulation, but by causing changes in the fluid on the cervix and changes in the lining of the uterus. Its long-term effects are not known, and it is not recommended for young women yet.

The "morning-after" pill *(diethylstilbestrol)* has recently been approved by the Food and Drug Administration for use only in emergencies (like rape). This pill is a *very* high dose of synthetic estrogen. It is taken for five days (or sometimes in a single dose) no more than twenty-four hours after intercourse. It prevents the fertilized egg from implanting in the uterus. The morning-after pill usually causes nausea and vomiting and doesn't always work. If it fails, you should have an abortion, since if the baby is female, there is a high risk that she (not you) will develop cancer of the vagina before she's twenty years old. Many doctors and others concerned with public health believe that diethylstilbestrol should never be used for any reason, because of the risks.

Rhythm

Rhythm is a method of birth control which involves neither mechanical nor chemical interference with reproduction. It is based on the fact that a woman is able to get pregnant for only a few days out of every month. What you have to do to use rhythm successfully is figure out when you normally ovulate. Then, you simply don't have intercourse around that time. Although it sounds simple, rhythm is the most complicated of the birth control methods.

If you want to use rhythm, you have to keep a record of your menstrual cycle (the number of days from the first day of one period to the first day of the next) for at least eight months and preferably for a year. Then, when you have all those numbers, you can begin to calculate.

SUBTRACT eighteen from the *shortest* cycle. This gives you your first "unsafe" day. For instance, if your shortest cycle in the year was twenty-five days, then the first unsafe day of any later cycle is day seven. Remember that you always count from the first day of your period.

Then SUBTRACT eleven from the *longest* cycle. This gives you your last unsafe day. So if your longest cycle was thirty-four days, your last unsafe day is twenty-three days after the start of your period. Thus, in this case, you are safe only from day one to day six of your cycle (which is probably while you have your period) and after the twenty-third day. This means you can't have intercourse from the seventh to the twenty-third day.

You can also figure out when you ovulate by keeping a temperature chart. Since your normal body temperature drops slightly when ovulation takes place and then rises one-half to one degree Fahrenheit, a chart will indicate when you have ovulated. The problem here is that the drop is often too small to be noticed, and by the time the rise takes place, you've already ovulated and may already be pregnant. To keep a chart, you have to take your temperature every morning *before* you get up, and record the results.

Aside from the difficulty of keeping accurate records, there are other problems with the rhythm method. Live sperm have been found on a woman's cervix up to a week after intercourse. Since the calculation of the "safe" period is based on the fact that sperm *usually* survive for only three days, you might still get pregnant from intercourse during the safe period, just because the sperm were hardier than the average.

Most women under the age of twenty-two have somewhat irregular menstrual cycles, and some women have irregular cycles all their lives. Ovulation can sometimes occur at unusual times during the cycle. Some women ovulate a few days earlier than average in the cycle; some a few days later. Once in a while, a woman may ovulate while she is menstruating. For this reason alone, rhythm is not usually recommended for young women. If you decide, however, that you want to use rhythm for religious or other reasons, you should get the advice of a doctor on the best way to proceed. In general, it is not a reliable method. And once you've carefully

˙calculated your safe period, you have to have perfect self-control about *never* having intercourse *except* during the safe period.

Some Methods That Don't Control Birth

Withdrawal, also known as "being careful," is the oldest known method of birth control. Unfortunately, it doesn't work very well, though it's better than nothing. Withdrawal means that the man pulls his penis out of the vagina before he ejaculates, so that, in theory, no sperm get into the vagina. However, there are sperm in the few drops of lubricating fluid that seep from the penis before the final ejaculation. Even this small number of sperm may cause a pregnancy. It is also really difficult for a man to withdraw just before orgasm, so he needs excellent self-control. The final problem is that since the sperm can move by themselves, it is possible for them to swim into the vagina if they are deposited near, though not in, it. There are cases of women who have never had complete intercourse but became pregnant from sperm ejaculated outside the vagina.

Douching (cleaning the vagina with a water or chemical solution spray) after intercourse is probably the worst "birth control" method you can use. Supposedly, to be effective, the douching must be done immediately after intercourse. "Immediately" means within seconds. However, douching after intercourse, no matter how soon you do it, may force the sperm *into* the uterus and may actually increase your chances of becoming pregnant. And there is really no way to get to the douche fast enough to be sure that no sperm are already in the uterus, where the douche won't touch them anyway. Using Coke as a douche will not prevent pregnancy, but *will* possibly cause a yeast infection in the vagina because of all the sugar in the Coke. (Sugar helps yeast to grow.)

Another popular but untrue idea is that if the woman doesn't have an orgasm, she can't get pregnant. Orgasm has *nothing* to do with pregnancy. And standing up during or after intercourse, so the sperm won't get into the uterus, doesn't work either. The sperm swim, and they can swim uphill.

Sterilization—The Final Control

Although sterilization is probably not something that you'll be considering for yourself for a while, you may hear your parents talking about it, or you may have read or heard about if from others. Sterilization is the permanent prevention of pregnancy by surgical means. Both men and women can be sterilized.

The most common technique of sterilization for women is called *tubal ligation,* or tying the Fallopian tubes. The woman is placed under general anesthesia (that is, she is put to sleep), and a small incision is made in the abdomen. Then each of the

Fallopian tubes is cut, and the ends are tied off. Women can also be sterilized by having the entire uterus removed. This procedure is called a *hysterectomy*. Hysterectomy is a much more serious operation than tubal ligation and should only be done when the uterus has been damaged somehow or

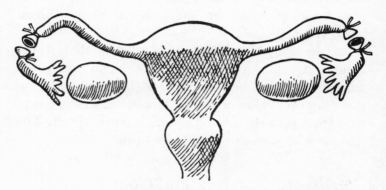

TUBAL LIGATION
(Sterilization of female)

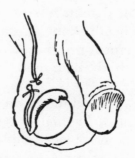

VASECTOMY
(Sterilization of male)

when there are tumors. It should never be done only to prevent future pregnancies.

Men are sterilized by a process called *vasectomy.* This is a simple procedure usually done in a doctor's office with local anesthesia. It involves a small incision in the scrotum, through which the vas deferens, which carries sperm from the testes to the penis, can be reached. The vas is cut, a section of it is removed, and the ends of the cut are closed. The man still ejaculates when he has an orgasm, since the sperm only make up about 10 percent of the ejaculatory fluid and everything but the sperm is still there.

Tubal ligation and vasectomy, since they don't interfere with the production of sperm, eggs, or hormones, do not have any effect on male or female physical characteristics or on sexual desire. People who have been sterilized have completely normal sexual relations, but they can't get pregnant or cause a pregnancy.

Some doctors and hospitals will not sterilize a person who is below a certain age (which varies from hospital to hospital) or who has not already had a certain number of children, unless there is evidence that a pregnancy would be fatal to the mother. Thus, a young couple who are sure that they want no children, or only one or two, may not be able to be sterilized until one of them is past thirty or thirty-five. Sterilization can occasionally be reversed by further surgery, but since you can't depend on that, it has to be considered permanent.

Anyone who is thinking about being sterilized, or whose doctor recommends it, must be fully informed of the risks involved in surgery. She must also be informed, in language she can understand, that sterilization means that she can never have a baby afterward. Too many women are pressured into being sterilized without clearly understanding the consequences.

8

When Birth Control Fails
What They Didn't Tell You in Biology 101

Any birth control method can fail. Even after sterilization, the tubes have been known to grow back together (although this is a very rare occurrence), and then pregnancy can occur. Of course, the more carefully and consistently you use whatever method you've chosen, the better your chances are of not becoming pregnant. But whether you're using birth control or not, if you've had intercourse and you miss a period, you have to consider the possibility that you may be pregnant.

When your period is late, it's perfectly natural to worry a lot and do nothing but hope that it will finally come. You keep running to the bathroom to see if you've got your period, and you keep looking

at the calendar and counting the days. If you keep
records of your cycle, you'll know within a few days
if you're late. If you didn't have intercourse during
the month, then you're probably not pregnant. Occasionally there are "false periods" in early pregnancy.
If you have a lighter than usual period with other
signs (fatigue, nausea, frequent urination), you
should suspect a pregnancy. (If there's no chance
that you're pregnant and you don't get your period,
assuming that it's fairly regular, you should see a
doctor to find out what is happening.) If there's any
possibility that you might be pregnant, then the
sooner you realize it and do something about it, the
better off you'll be. If your period is only five to ten
days late, you can go to a doctor or clinic and get
progesterone, which will bring on your period *only
if you are not pregnant.* It won't cause an abortion if
you are. If you don't get your period after taking
progesterone, you are probably pregnant, and you
should immediately get a pregnancy test.

Getting a Pregnancy Test

There are lots of things that can delay your period.
Stress (and that includes worry about being pregnant), a cold or other illness, emotional shock, or
traveling can all throw you off schedule. If your
period is delayed more than ten days longer than
your longest previous cycle, the time has come to get
a pregnancy test. If you live in a large city, that's no

problem, no matter what your age. There are always ads in underground or college newspapers telling you where you can get a free or inexpensive urine test. The test itself usually takes only a couple of minutes. Hospital prenatal clinics always do pregnancy tests. In most areas, Planned Parenthood clinics not only will do the test but have doctors who will examine you to determine how far along you are if the test is positive. If the test is negative (meaning that you're not pregnant) and you don't get a period within a week, you must have another test.

If You're Pregnant

Once you know that you're pregnant, try to stay calm. There is plenty of help available to you. And since you've been acting responsibly so far, this is not the time to panic. You have to face up to the fact that you *are* pregnant, so that you can do something about it. Not admitting it to yourself, or hoping that it will just go away, is no solution. Eventually it's going to be impossible to hide, and the sooner you take action the more choices you have and the better you'll feel. If possible, talk things over with the boy who's responsible. He may not be very helpful, he may even be nasty, but it's his problem too. You may want him to help pay for an abortion, or help you figure out what to do, or be with you when and if you tell your parents.

One of the hardest things to do, and the thing that

most pregnant girls worry most about, is telling parents. *Most* parents, after some initial bad reaction, take the news pretty well and are inclined to be helpful. Some take it badly and never let you forget it. If you're planning to have the baby, or if you're under seventeen and want an abortion, they're almost certainly going to have to know you're pregnant. You may find it easiest to tell someone you trust first and then have that person with you when you tell your parents.

In all large cities and in many smaller ones, there are counseling services for women with unplanned pregnancies. The counselors (usually women) are there to help you decide what you want to do and to help you do whatever you decide. They won't be surprised or shocked, no matter what your story is or how young you are, and they won't force you to do anything you don't want to do. The decision is often not an easy one, and someone who has experience and knows all the possible choices can be of great help.

If there is a women's center in your community, it probably offers pregnancy counseling or can direct you to someone who does. If not, look in local underground or campus newspapers for anything called a pregnancy counseling service, abortion counseling service, or women's health group. This service should be free or *very* low cost (some groups ask for a contribution). If someone asks for twenty-five dollars or more, try to find another service. If you can't find a counseling service locally, you can call the Clergy Consultation Service. This is a nationwide network of clergymen who will help you decide what you want to do about your pregnancy. They will help you make any necessary arrangements (like setting up an appointment at an abortion clinic or maternity home) and will help you tell your parents if necessary. Look them up in your local phone book. If they're not listed, call 212-254-6230 (that's in New York City). The telephone is answered twenty-four hours a day, and they will direct you to someone near where you live. Planned Parenthood clinics in most areas also offer pregnancy counseling. There are Planned Parenthood clinics in all cities and in a lot of towns.

Once you know that you're pregnant, you have several choices. You can decide to get married. You can decide not to get married but to have the baby. Then you have the further choice of keeping it or giving it up for adoption. Or you can decide to have an abortion. But you have to do something. ABOVE ALL, DON'T TRY TO ABORT YOURSELF OR HAVE A FRIEND HELP ABORT YOU. You can kill yourself or make yourself permanently sterile that way. And you'll undoubtedly wind up in a hospital and then your parents will find out about it anyway.

Having an Abortion

If you find yourself pregnant when you don't want to be, I think your best choice is to have an abortion. Abortion is now supposed to be available every-

where. The United States Supreme Court decided in
January 1973 that states cannot restrict abortion at
all if the woman is less than twelve weeks pregnant.
Up to twenty-four weeks, abortion is still supposed
to be available, but the states then have the right to
restrict it to hospitals and can make other regulations concerning the medical procedures. If your life
or health is in danger because of the pregnancy, you
may still get an abortion after twenty-four weeks.
This is now technically the law everywhere. However, in some states, because of laws still on the
books or because of the attitudes of doctors in that
state, it is practically impossible to get an abortion.
If you want an abortion and don't know where to go,
the Clergy Consultation Service or the nearest
Planned Parenthood branch will be able to help you.
It has always been the case that when women are
prevented from having legal abortions, they will
find ways of getting illegal abortions, which are
much more dangerous. There should no longer be
any reason for a woman to have to risk her life or her
health having an illegal abortion.

A legal early abortion performed by a trained person under sterile conditions is one of the least dangerous medical procedures you can have done. The
risk of complications from a legal abortion is less
than the risk of complications in a full-term pregnancy.

Contrary to what you may hear from people who
are opposed to abortion, most women who have
abortions don't feel guilty or depressed or anything

but relieved afterward. Before abortion was legalized, when millions of married and unmarried women had illegal abortions anyway, the fear of being discovered, the underground nature of the whole business, and the fact that abortion was never talked about openly gave many women negative feelings about it. After five years of legal abortion in New York State, it has been found that only rarely does a woman report feeling guilty after an abortion. Some women do get depressed for a day or so, but this is usually the result of the sudden drop in hormone levels and not an emotional reaction to the fact of the abortion. Every abortion facility should have counselors available to explain the abortion procedure, to discuss birth control, and to discuss your feelings about the abortion if you want to talk about them. The counselor should stay with you throughout the procedure if it is done under local anesthesia.

Although abortion can be performed at any time, the earlier you have one the better. Up to twelve weeks of pregnancy, the procedure can usually be done in a doctor's office or a clinic where you don't have to stay overnight. The abortion, at this stage, is usually done by a procedure called *vacuum aspiration* or *suction curettage*. The cervix is gradually stretched and the contents of the uterus are very gently withdrawn through a narrow tube attached to a suction device. This can be done while you are awake. The dilation (opening) of the cervix is usually somewhat painful, rather like menstrual cramps, and so a local anesthetic (like Novocaine) is injected near the cervix. Cramps usually last up to one hour after the abortion. If you are very tense about the abortion, you may want to have it done under general anesthesia, which means you are put to sleep for the few minutes that it takes. The vacuum aspiration itself takes about five minutes. With time allowed for tests (blood tests, venereal disease tests, etc.), counseling, and about an hour in the recovery room, you should be in the clinic for three to four hours altogether, if you have had local anesthesia. With general anesthesia, though you wake up within a few minutes after the procedure, you have to stay at the clinic for three to four hours after the abortion. So if you have general anesthesia, you will probably be at the clinic or hospital for six to eight hours.

A new procedure called *menstrual extraction* is sometimes done within the week or two after a missed period. It is very much like the vacuum aspiration technique described above, but different instruments are used and the cervix is stretched very little. Local anesthesia is used. After the procedure, the tissue removed from the uterus is examined to determine whether the woman was pregnant or not, since menstrual extraction is often done before a woman is pregnant long enough to have a positive pregnancy test. However, if you aren't pregnant to begin with, then menstrual extraction is just an unnecessary medical procedure, and some doctors believe it should never be done unless the pregnancy test is positive.

If you are between twelve and fourteen weeks pregnant, a *dilatation and curettage* (D&C) is done. In some places, the D&C is the standard method for all abortions up to fourteen weeks. General anesthesia is usually used for a D&C. The cervix is gently dilated, using a series of cigar-shaped metal tubes (as in the vacuum aspiration procedure), and then the uterus is gently scraped with a metal instrument called a *curette*. If you have a D&C, you usually have to stay overnight in the hospital.

There is no safe way to do an abortion between fourteen and sixteen weeks of pregnancy. The uterus has become too soft and thin for a D&C to be done safely, and the uterus is not yet large enough for a saline induction.

For pregnancies over sixteen weeks, the usual abortion technique is a *saline induction.* A small patch of the abdomen is anesthetized with Novocaine or something similar, and some of the fluid in the uterus is withdrawn through a needle which is inserted into the uterus through the abdomen. The fluid is then replaced with a sugar or salt (saline) solution. This procedure is not painful. Within six to forty-eight hours, contractions begin, and a miscarriage is induced. These contractions may hurt, and pain-killing drugs can be given. Occasionally, it is necessary to give a second dose of sugar or salt solution to get the process started. This technique can only be done in a hospital, and most hospitals require that you stay until the miscarriage is complete.

This means that you may be in the hospital up to three days. In a few places, doctors are using substances called *prostaglandins* to start the miscarriage.

Very occasionally, a late abortion is done by an operation called *hysterotomy* (not to be confused with hysterectomy, which is the removal of the uterus). A hysterotomy is a major operation, in which an incision is made through the abdomen into the uterus and the fetus is taken out. Hysterotomy should only be done when there is a medical reason for not doing a saline induction.

Early abortions are simple procedures and should be relatively inexpensive. In New York, the cost of a vacuum aspiration abortion is usually between $90 and $200, and most of the clinics can sometimes arrange an even lower price (like $25) or time payments, if money is a problem. An abortion done in a hospital, in New York or anywhere else, is of course more expensive. A D&C can cost $200 to $300. A saline induction can cost up to $1,000, though they can be found for as low as $250. Some hospitals will give you a flat rate for a saline induction, and others charge according to how long you are actually in the hospital. SHOP AROUND if you possibly can when you're planning to get an abortion. Ask the doctor, counselor, or clinic for names of more than one place, and find out all you can before you decide where to go. A few extra phone calls may save you several hundred dollars in the long run. Paying more for an abortion doesn't usually mean that you're getting a safer abortion; it just means that the doctor or hospital is making more profit.

If you have problems once you get to the clinic or hospital for an abortion, you should definitely report back to whoever referred you. Whether the problem is a medical complication or dissatisfaction with the counseling you received or with the fees or anything, the person who referred you should be told. Don't just forget about it. Abortion is big business these days, and we all deserve the best possible treatment. By reporting problems, you can help to insure that other women will have better service.

If You Decide to Have the Baby

Having the baby and raising it alone is a very difficult thing to do. And you must be prepared to be the one who raises the baby—for about twenty years. You can't depend on your mother to do the job. She probably figures that she's through with babies and may well have other plans for herself. Some women are successful at raising their children alone. Others have tried it for a while and then have had to make the difficult decision to give the child up anyway. If you're thinking of raising a baby alone, talk to a woman who's done it, either one who's been alone from the beginning or one who later separated from the child's father. She should be able to give you practical advice and help you make a decision.

If you're going to raise your baby alone, you'll have to figure out how you'll support yourself and a child. The father has a legal responsibility to contribute to a child's support, and you can get a court to set the amount of money he has to give you. The burden of getting him to pay, however, will fall mainly on you. If he refuses to pay, you have to find him and bring him into court by having a summons issued. In court he'll be threatened with jail if he doesn't pay what he owes. If he's still in school, the court can't order him to pay very much, so the main responsibility will still be yours. You can usually go on welfare if you're single and have a baby, but you should check the regulations where you live before you count on that. Welfare doesn't give you very much, and you may find that it's not enough for you to get along on.

Before you decide to have the baby, whether or not you get married, you have to take into account what having a child will mean for your life. A baby is not a toy. It is a completely helpless human being who will be dependent on you for everything, for a long time, whether you feel like dealing with it or not. Having brought a child into the world, you and the baby's father are responsible for making that child's life as good as it can be. You can't decide to sleep late and ignore the baby. You can't just take a day off. You won't be able to go out with friends before making arrangements for the baby. You won't be able to do much but take care of the baby for a long time, unless you can pay baby-sitters, and even then you're still responsible for making sure that the sitter is taking good care of your child.

Having the baby and giving it up for adoption is another possibility. If you decide that that's what you want to do, check out the adoption services in your area carefully. There are public (often Department of Welfare) agencies and private ones. It should be possible for you to get your medical expenses paid by the agency, and they may also be able to make arrangements for you to go to a maternity home, if that's what you want to do. In most states, once you sign the papers after the baby is born, you can't get the child back. People who adopt children really want them, so you can be sure that your baby will be loved and well cared for.

If you are certain that you do *not* want an abortion, you can contact an organization called Birthright, which has branches in major cities. Most Birthright counselors do not approve of abortion under any circumstances, even in cases of rape or when the baby is sure to be defective. They can arrange for you to live with a family outside your community while you are pregnant. You will be expected to baby-sit and do housework for the family. If you are sent to a family you don't like, you have the right to leave. They will arrange for another family. Toward the end of the pregnancy, you can go to a maternity home. You will be expected to pay something toward the cost of that. Birthright will also provide counseling throughout the pregnancy and will arrange for the adoption of the baby if you don't want to keep it.

Pregnancy by itself should not be a reason to get married. Getting married just because you're pregnant usually means that your chances of having a good marriage are slim. If you were already planning to marry the boy involved and you've considered what marriage to him would be like, if you've figured out how you'll support yourselves and a child and considered how a child fits in with both your plans for education or a career, you may make a success of it. However, if you haven't answered all those questions in a realistic way, you're probably in for some nasty surprises. Things won't just work out, even if you love each other.

Above all, if you suspect that you are pregnant, have a test. And if you *are* pregnant, tell someone immediately. If you're going to have the baby, you need to get medical care as early as possible in the pregnancy, so you can have a healthy pregnancy and a healthy baby. If you're not going to have the baby, then the sooner you have the abortion and get it over with, the better you're going to feel. Too many women put off doing something about a pregnancy until it's too late to do *anything* except have the baby. The pregnancy won't just go away, no matter how hard you hope that it will. It's going to stay there and become more and more obvious. You won't have an easier time telling your parents when you're six months pregnant than you will when you're two months pregnant. So instead of walking around scared and worried and wondering, make a decision and act on it immediately.

9

Venereal Disease, Vaginal Infections, and Other Things
What They Didn't Tell You in Biology 101

Most people have by now heard that venereal disease is the most serious and widespread epidemic in North America. More people will get gonorrhea this year than any other disease that is passed from one person to another, except the common cold. In spite of the publicity about the epidemic, the rate continues to rise. There are several reasons for the increase in VD: inadequate health care, the lack of massive testing programs, confusion about the symptoms, and the fear and guilt that many people have about VD. On top of all that, most people are still taught to believe that VD is some kind of punishment for sexual freedom. The highest rates of VD in North America occur among young people and poor people—those who have the least access to good health care.

The VD problem for women is complicated by the fact that there are several different infections of the vagina which have symptoms that are much like the symptoms of VD, and by the fact that women may get VD and have no outward signs of it for a long time. For this reason, it is important for any woman who is having sexual relations to have tests for gonorrhea and syphilis at least once a year. If you are having sex with several different people, or if you are having sex with a person who has several different partners, it's a good idea to get a test at least twice a year. Very often, a woman only finds out that she might have VD when a man with whom she's had sex tells her that he has it. Although a woman can have syphilis or gonorrhea for a long time without noticing it, both diseases are very serious and can cause terrible problems.

If you think you have VD, the worst thing you can do is sit around and worry about it. The hardest part is the initial step of finding out where to get a test and making the appointment. If you do have VD, the treatment is simple and quick. And if you don't have it, you'll be able to stop worrying.

Gonorrhea

Although gonorrhea is considered medically less serious than syphilis because it doesn't kill, it is a much more common disease and is the one you're most likely to get. You can't get gonorrhea (or syphilis, for that matter) from toilet seats, towels, doorknobs, or kissing. The germ that causes gonorrhea (called a *gonococcus*) cannot live for more than a very few seconds outside the human body. Therefore, it can be transmitted *only* by direct contact with the infected parts of another person. The usual way to get gonorrhea is by sexual intercourse or close contact with the sex organs of an infected person. It can be picked up only in the genitals, the mouth, or the anus. Since the gonococcus only grows well on mucous membranes, such as those that line the vagina, you can't get it by touching an infected penis with your hand.

The real danger of gonorrhea lies in the fact that 80 percent of the women who have it show no symptoms until the disease and the damage it does are well advanced. Thus, we are too often dependent on the honesty of the men we're sleeping with to tell us that we may have the disease. Gonorrhea in women usually attacks the cervix first. Sometimes there is an irritating discharge from the vagina a few days after infection. The discharge will be yellow or greenish. There are other infections which produce a discharge that looks the same. The clear or whitish discharge that occurs normally is not a sign of disease. However, a yellow or green or thick, heavy white discharge, though it may signal an infection other than gonorrhea, is always cause for a visit to the doctor.

A gonorrhea infection can be spread from the vagina to the urethra. If this happens, there will be pain and burning when you urinate. Early gonorrhea may also cause low backache or mild pain in the lower abdomen.

If it isn't treated, the infection travels up into the uterus (where it doesn't grow very well) and into the Fallopian tubes, where it causes *salpingitis,* which means infection of the Fallopian tubes. Pus forms in the tubes, and the infection can spread from the ends of the tubes onto the ovaries and into the pelvic cavity. At this stage, the condition is called *pelvic inflammatory disease* (PID). The outward signs of PID are fever, severe pain in the abdomen, nausea, and headache. The same symptoms can be produced by appendicitis. Sometimes the symptoms of PID are quite mild and it is mistaken for a "virus." The fever may be only a little above normal, and the pain may not be severe. If the disease is left untreated, scar tissue will eventually form in the tubes and on the ovaries. If the tubes are completely blocked by scar tissue, conception is not possible and the woman is totally sterile. This is the most serious result of gonorrhea for women. If the tube is only partly closed, fertilization of the egg in the tube may still be possible because the sperm, which are very small, may be able to get through whatever opening is left. However, that opening may be too small for the much larger egg to proceed down the tube. The fertilized egg will then implant in the Fallopian tube instead of in the uterus. This is called a *tubal* or *ectopic pregnancy.* (You can also have a tubal pregnancy for reasons other than gonorrhea.) The tube, which can't stretch very much, will eventually burst from the pressure of the fetus growing in it, usually within six to twelve weeks of pregnancy, causing severe internal bleeding. Immediate medical care is necessary to save the woman's life if this happens.

Since both the early and the late symptoms of gonorrhea can be confused with the signs of other diseases, and since so many women have no symptoms at all, you can only be sure that you don't have gonorrhea by having a test for it. Of course, if a boy you're having intercourse with tells you that he has gonorrhea, you must go for testing immediately. If you're having sexual relations even occasionally, you should be going for a gynecological checkup once a year. When you do, you should ask to have a gonorrhea test done. The test should be done on everyone, and you shouldn't have to ask for it, but often you do. The doctor should take a culture, by removing some of the fluid on the cervix and the urethra with a cotton swab and then smearing it on a special substance where any gonorrhea germs in it will grow. The culture is sent to a lab where it is kept for several days and then examined.

To diagnose gonorrhea in a man, it's usually sufficient for the doctor to take some of the discharge from the penis, smear it on a glass slide, and immediately look at it under a microscope. The smear technique is rarely useful for diagnosing gonorrhea in women. Insist that the doctor do a *culture,* not a smear. If he won't, any public health station will do a test for free.

About 90 percent of the men who have gonorrhea show symptoms within three to five days after infection. The first sign is usually a thin, clear discharge from the end of the penis. Within a few days, the discharge becomes thicker and turns white or yellow. Urination becomes extremely painful, and it is the painful urination that usually gets the man to a doctor. If the disease is not treated, the pain during urination will eventually disappear as the infection travels up the reproductive tract. Untreated gonorrhea in a man can infect the testes, the prostate, or the tubes that lead from one to the other. The infection may cause scarring of the tubes, which may close them, leaving the man sterile.

If you think or suspect that you have gonorrhea, you must get tested and treated as soon as possible. Minors (people under eighteen) can now be tested and treated for VD without their parents' consent in every state. To find out where to go for testing and treatment in your area, you can call Operation Venus, a VD information service set up by and for teenagers. The number (toll free) is 800-523-1885 from anywhere except Pennsylvania. From Pennsylvania, it's 1-800-462-4966. In the Philadelphia area, the number is 767-6969. They won't ask your name or anything about you. They just give out information.

Gonorrhea is easily cured with penicillin. However, you must be tested before you're given the penicillin to make sure that you have gonorrhea. The best kind of penicillin to cure gonorrhea is not the best kind to treat syphilis. You should be asked to return in a week or two for retesting. Occasionally, one dose of penicillin isn't enough to cure the disease. Avoid sexual intercourse until you're sure that you're cured. If you're allergic to penicillin, you will be treated with tetracycline or erythromycin. Tetracycline must not be taken by pregnant women, so if you're pregnant, be sure to tell the doctor.

Syphilis

Syphilis is an extremely serious disease, but it can be easily cured at any stage. The disease is especially difficult to detect without a test because its symptoms can be confused with those of other diseases and because the signs of the disease come and go by themselves. But syphilis remains in the body unless it's treated, and years after it was first picked up, the really severe effects show up. Among these are heart disease, paralysis, and insanity. It is estimated that there are about five hundred thousand people who have syphilis but don't know it. Some of these cases will be found when the person involved has a blood test for syphilis, which is required by all states before marriage, when entering a hospital, or when joining the armed forces. In addition, some people are cured of syphilis that they didn't know they had when they're given antibiotics to cure something else.

Three to four weeks after sexual intercourse with a person who is infected with syphilis, a sore called a *chancre* (pronounced "shanker") appears at the site of the infection. This is usually on the genitals, but may appear in the mouth or throat if that part of the body was in contact with the infected person's genitals. Since the organism that causes syphilis (*Treponema pallidum*) dies on contact with dry air or soap and water, it is practically impossible for it to be transmitted other than by sexual intercourse. You don't get it from toilet seats, towels, etc. In women, the chancre usually appears on the cervix or inside the vagina, although it may appear on the lips of the vagina. Since the chancre is usually painless, it probably won't be noticed if it is inside. In men, the chancre usually appears at or near the tip of the penis, and is therefore noticeable. Any person who develops a syphilitic chancre and doesn't tell his or her sexual partners should be expelled from the human race. The chancre, when it first appears, looks like a dull red pimple. It soon opens and some fluid may ooze from it or it may have a crusty scab. If not treated, it goes away by itself in one to five weeks. Sometimes it leaves a scar, sometimes not. Although the infected person has no symptoms, he or she can still infect someone else.

A month or so (sometimes as long as six months) after the chancre begins to develop, a skin rash de-

velops. The appearance of the rash varies widely
from person to person. The only thing that can be
said definitely is that it doesn't hurt or itch. The rash
may be mild or severe, widespread or local. Sometimes it appears on the palms of the hands or the
soles of the feet, and this is important because most
other rashes don't affect those areas. If the person
gets antibiotic treatment at this stage, the disease
clears up quickly and there are no lasting effects. If
the condition isn't treated, the rash and the feeling
of general bad health (headaches, nausea, fever) that
sometimes accompanies it will go away. The disease
itself hasn't gone away, however, but has only gone
into its latent stage.

During the latent stage of syphilis, some people
get a relapse of the chancre or the rash. Others have
no symptoms at all. A person who has latent syphilis
can infect others for about a year through cuts or
open areas on his or her body. But to be infected by a
person with latent syphilis, you'd have to get your
mouth or genitals in contact with the cut or sore.
After that, the disease is no longer contagious—with
one important exception: a woman with untreated
syphilis will give it to her unborn child, who may
die shortly before or after birth or be brain-damaged.

All pregnant women in North America are given a
blood test for syphilis as soon as possible after a
pregnancy is confirmed. If the mother is found to
have syphilis and is treated for it before the six-
teenth or eighteenth week of pregnancy, there is no
chance of damage to the baby. That's one of the

reasons why it's so important to see a doctor early in your pregnancy.

Years after the first infection, the late symptoms of syphilis show up. Although the disease can still be cured at this stage, the damage already done by it usually can't be corrected. The disease can infect the heart and major blood vessels, which is usually fatal. Or the brain and spinal cord can be affected, which may cause paralysis or insanity.

Any sore on the genitals, although it may not be syphilis, is enough reason to see a doctor. If you suspect that you might have syphilis, or if someone you've had intercourse with tells you that he has it, then you must have a blood test. The test may not show a positive result for four to six weeks after you've been exposed, so if it's negative (which means that you don't have syphilis) you should go back for retesting a few weeks later. Operation Venus will tell you where you can be tested and treated near your home.

Syphilis is best treated with one injection of a slow-acting type of penicillin, which is absorbed in small amounts over a period of a week or two. You should be tested for both syphillis and gonorrhea before the treatment is started, because the kind of penicillin that cures gonorrhea won't always clear up syphilis. If you are allergic to penicillin, you'll be given tetracycline or erythromycin.

Once you've been treated for syphilis, you must go back several times for reexamination and testing. You should be rechecked one month after the initial treatment and then once every three months for the next year. Although this may be inconvenient, it should be worth it when you consider the consequences of an untreated syphilis infection.

When you go to a VD clinic, someone is going to ask you for a list of all the people you've had sex with recently. All private doctors are supposed to get this information too, although many of them don't. The people you name will be contacted in confidence by the Public Health Service and asked to come in for testing. Being asked to give names is often embarrassing. And, unfortunately, in some places the VD clinics are so swamped with cases that they can't track the people down anyway. It's very important that, once you know you have a venereal disease, you *must* tell your sexual partners. That's sometimes not easy, but if you've been having sex with someone, you have a responsibility to him or her. The consequences of untreated VD are so serious that it can't be ignored in the hope that it will go away by itself and that your partners won't eventually find out that you gave it to them.

Vaginal Infections

The normal healthy vagina contains several different kinds of germs, and these help to keep the vagina slightly acid. Healthy vaginal walls produce a moist secretion which may be clear or slightly milky. The amount of the secretions varies during the menstrual cycle, often being heaviest just before or after menstruation or around the time of ovulation. It is also heavier during pregnancy and when you are sexually excited. If the discharge doesn't cause any discomfort and doesn't have a strong odor, it is nothing to worry about.

Anything that disturbs the normal kind and quantity of germs and secretions in the vagina can make you more likely to get an infection. Very often, if you're taking antibiotics to cure an infection somewhere else in your body, the antibiotic will kill off the germs that occur normally in the vagina. That will give the yeasts that also occur normally in the vagina and that are kept in control by the germs a chance to grow. So you may wind up with a yeast infection. Douching or using vaginal sprays will also destroy the healthy balance in the vagina and make you more likely to get infections. Birth control pills also cause changes in the vagina which make it easy for the yeasts to grow, and women who take pills sometimes get infections that are so persistent they have to stop taking the pills before the infection can be cured. There are three main types of *vaginitis,* or vaginal infection: *yeast, Trichomonas,* and *nonspecific.*

Yeast (also called *monilia, candida,* or *fungus*) causes a white discharge, which may be thin, or thick and cheeselike. The discharge smells like yeast and causes itching and irritation. If you look inside the vagina with a hand mirror, you will usually see white patches on the walls of the vagina if you have a yeast infection.

Yeast infections are usually quickly and easily cured. If you're pretty sure you have a yeast infection (if the discharge is white), you can try douching twice a week with two teaspoons of baking soda in a quart of warm water. If the condition hasn't cleared up in a week, see a doctor. A doctor will prescribe Monostat cream or tablets of Mycostatin, which are placed inside the vagina every morning and night for ten days to two weeks. Either one has to be used for the full time to make sure that the infection is really gone. The discharge and itching usually stop within a few days. Desitin ointment or powder applied on the outside can help to relieve the itch, as will a cool bath with baking soda in the water. Intercourse isn't dangerous when you have a monilia infection, but it may be painful because it increases the irritation.

Since the yeast grows in warm, damp places, any clothing that keeps the air from circulating around the genitals can encourage its growth. If you have a yeast infection (or tend to get a lot of them), it may help to switch from nylon to cotton underpants, which allow more circulation of air. Tights, pantyhose, tight pants, and nylon or latex bathing suits can also make you more uncomfortable.

Trichomonas (not trichinosis, which you can get from undercooked pork) is caused by a microscopic one-celled animal. A *Trichomonas* infection causes a yellow or greenish yellow (not white) discharge which may be foamy or slimy and which causes irritation and itching. For suspected *Tricho-*

monas, douche twice weekly with two teaspoons of vinegar in a quart of warm water. If the infection persists, see your doctor. If you have an infection which you think is *Trichomonas,* it's advisable to get a test for gonorrhea, since the early symptoms are similar. A doctor will prescribe a pill called Flagyl, which is taken by mouth and usually works very well. It is taken for ten days, three times a day. Drinking any kind of alcohol, even beer or wine, while you're taking Flagyl can cause severe nausea and vomiting. If the infection isn't cleared up in ten days, you have to go back to the doctor. He will either prescribe more Flagyl or another medication which is placed directly inside the vagina. Since Flagyl kills other things besides the *Trichomonas,* you may get a yeast infection as soon as the *Trichomonas* is cleared up. Anyone you have sex with regularly while you have a *Trichomonas* infection should also take Flagyl. Although a man won't have any symptoms himself, he may be carrying the organisms and can reinfect you. Then you'll have to start treatment all over again. Men can transmit *Trichomonas* from one woman to another. If *you* get a *Trichomonas* infection, it is his responsibility to tell any other women he's having sex with that they may be infected.

Nonspecific vaginitis is caused by bacteria. There is itching and swelling of the vagina and a white or yellow discharge that may be streaked with blood. The usual treatment is with sulfa drugs, if you're not allergic to them, in cream or suppositories (tablets placed in the vagina). If you can't take sulfa drugs, other kinds of suppositories or douches will be prescribed. Whatever you're given, follow the doctor's instructions carefully, and make sure that you understand them before you leave the office or clinic. Nonspecific infections sometimes take a long time to be cured.

There are germs and other organisms in the intestinal tract that can cause yeast or bacterial infections if they are spread to the vagina. Therefore, it is important that nothing that has touched your feces be allowed to come into contact with your vagina. If you have anal sex (where the penis is in your rectum), it is most important that the man wash his penis thoroughly with soap and water before putting it into your vagina. After going to the bathroom, always wipe yourself from front to back. Healthy urine is germfree, and so won't hurt you if it gets near or into the vagina. Germs from the anus can be spread to the vagina on a sanitary pad, where they grow very well in the blood that's there. So you are safer using tampons, especially if you get a lot of infections.

Washing the outer genitals daily with soap and water is usually enough to prevent an infection from taking hold. Changing your underwear daily is also important. Monilia and *Trichomonas* can both be picked up from toilet seats, towels, and washcloths, if these have been used by an infected person and not washed.

Cystitis, or infection of the bladder, is usually caused by germs from the rectum or vagina getting into the bladder. There is a burning sensation when you urinate, and you may feel that you want to urinate very frequently. There may also be blood in the urine. The usual treatment is with Gantrisin (a sulfa drug) or, in cases that are resistant to Gantrisin, with tetracycline. Gantrisin turns your urine bright orange, so don't be concerned if that happens.

Herpes sores look like cold sores, except that they appear on the genitals. They are caused by a virus and go away by themselves. However, if you get a sore and there is *any* chance that you've been exposed to syphilis, get a blood test. If you get herpes sores repeatedly, you should report this to your doctor.

Crabs are tiny animals called lice, that look like crabs when seen under a magnifying glass. They are usually found in the pubic hair, although they can get into other body hair as well. They bite and suck blood. They are *very* annoying. They can be passed on by your sexual partners, and also by sharing beds or towels. If you get crabs (you will see them as little white spots in your pubic hair), wash the whole area with Kwell cream, lotion, or shampoo, which you can get from the drugstore without a prescription. Wash all the bed linen, towels, and underwear that you've used, and don't let anyone else use them until you're certain the crabs are gone.

10

Parents

There are lots of books for parents about how to "handle" kids, but unfortunately, there aren't books for kids on how to handle parents. There are, however, some basic things you can try which may make it easier for you to "handle" your parents. The first thing to do, if you can, is to figure out what *they* are doing. Some parents have a "method" for raising their kids and try to stick to that method all the time. If they do have a method, that makes them easier in some ways for you to deal with, since you generally know what to expect from them. Other parents improvise from one situation to the next, which makes it harder for you to figure out in advance what they're going to do next. But in general you know by now whether your parents are fair or unfair, whether they're strict or easygoing, whether they're pleased or frightened by signs of your independence, and whether or not they can be reasoned with.

When you were a very small child, it probably seemed to you that your parents knew everything. You realize as you get older that they don't know everything and that at times they're not very sure of themselves. It's as hard for them to see you objectively as it is for you to see them objectively, and your dealings with one another are not always completely rational. By the time you're a teenager, you and your parents have a long and complicated relationship behind you, and you've developed patterns in relating with one another that may be difficult to break. You may be guilty of playing one parent off against the other, or always going along with what they want, or never going along with what they want. Patterns are individual, and it's good to see if you can discover what yours and your parents' are. Once you do recognize them, you'll be able to decide whether or not that's really the way you want to act. Until you recognize your own patterns, you have no chance of changing them.

If everything that happens in your family is the occasion for a fight between you and your parents, the three of you have already gotten yourselves into a useless way of behaving toward one another. Every good relationship includes some amount of conflict. But that conflict doesn't have to be in the form of screaming arguments, although these can sometimes be useful too.

If you get into a fight with your parents over every little thing, you may be disagreeing with them just for the sake of disagreeing. You're not thinking things through, and are assuming that they are always wrong. But that's really impossible. There are bound to be some things that you all do agree on, and it can only help to stop and try to figure out what those things are. It can't be very pleasant to fight all the time. It's natural for some of us, when we're angry about one thing, to pick a fight about something else. While it may be natural, it won't get you very far toward solving the problem that's making you angry in the first place. If you're furious with your mother because she won't let you go out on Saturday night, it's not going to help you much to pick a fight with her over who's going to do the dinner dishes. You may feel better for a little while because you released some of your feelings, but your problem about Saturday night still won't be solved. You'll also find that, even after the fight over the dishes, you're still angry. If you take on the real issue and let her know exactly how you feel about going out on Saturday night and why, perhaps you have a chance of working out a compromise.

At the other end of things, if you always go along with what your parents want, you've gotten yourself into an equally bad pattern. You're assuming that *they* are always right. That's impossible too. You'll have to gather up your courage and start telling them when you really disagree with something. It will get easier the more often you do it. Even when all the logical arguments seem to be on their side, your *feel-*

ings about a situation still count. If you are hurt or
angry or disappointed, or if you feel that something's unfair to you, those feelings *should* make a
difference to your parents. If you've been going
along with them without questioning for a long
time, it isn't likely that you will suddenly go over-
board in asserting your rights or wishes or feelings.
Don't worry about being too assertive. If you overdo
it, someone will tell you and you can deal with it
then.

Getting What You Want—Or What You Need

Very few parents are going to let you do everything you want to. That's a fact you simply have to
face. And the fact is that they do have the legal right
to make you do what they want. You are probably
financially dependent on them and, whatever your
age, if you have to count on someone to house and
feed you and pay your expenses, that someone can
exercise control over what you do. Your parents have
a legal responsibility to care for you, and that responsibility extends to behavior as well as to taking
care of your physical needs.

You can't do everything that you want to do, but
it's the rare set of parents who will refuse everything
you want to do. *You* have to decide what's most
important to you and, if you think what you want is
reasonable, go after that. Give in on the things that

you don't care about so much. You *can* bargain with
most parents. If you want to stay out later than usual
next weekend, then you may be able to trade that off
for extra time spent taking care of your little brother
or an extra turn doing the dishes. First you have to
be able to decide what's important to you. It may be
that nothing in the world would be worth having to
spend extra time with your brother. So then maybe
there's something else you can do. Or maybe you'll
decide that staying out late isn't important enough to
take on extra work for it.

There really isn't any point in making an issue of
every little thing that comes up. If you keep a sense
of proportion about what is important and what
isn't, your parents just might respond in kind. No
parents are always reasonable, any more than you
are, but most parents respond well if you treat them
right.

Some of the things that can make parents unreasonable have nothing to do with you. Your parents
have certain memories (which are not always accurate) of what it was like when they grew up. Whenever that was, things are different now, and they may
not realize exactly what that means. The things they
say to you may have made sense for them twenty or
thirty years ago, but they may be wrong now. It's
also probably true that your parents have a particular and perhaps limited view of who you really are.
Someone who sees you only in school could probably describe you to your parents, and your parents

wouldn't always recognize that you were being described. Of course, everyone acts differently in different situations, but your parents still remember you (and sometimes treat you) as a small child who was completely dependent on them, while your friends in school don't. So your parents may insist on treating you like a child when that's not necessary, and then, annoyingly, just when you're not feeling very sure of yourself about something, they'll want to treat you like a grown-up.

You know that it can sometimes be important to you to look like you know what you're doing even when you really don't. Some of us seem to suffer from that tendency worse than others, but almost everyone tries, at least once in a while, to look together when they don't feel that way at all. Your parents do it too. Being a parent is often difficult, and you can be absolutely sure that, no matter how they try to make it look, they don't always know what they're doing, or how to react, or when to say yes and when to say no. In general, most parents try to do what they think is best. They want to see you turn out okay, be happy, and (sometimes more important than it should be) not be a disgrace to them. Most parents are not trying to be nasty. If you can keep that in mind, you have a chance of persuading them to do things differently.

Making your parents change their minds about how to treat you puts an enormous burden on you. When you want to do something and they say no, your reaction is probably to get furious, whether you show it or not. And if you know that there's nothing wrong with what you want to do, you have a right to be furious. (Of course, if you want to use the car when you don't know how to drive, or don't have a license, it's unrealistic to be surprised when they won't let you.) However, yelling at your mother because you feel that she's being unreasonable may not be the most productive thing for you to do. You probably don't react very well when someone yells at you, and you shouldn't expect your mother to either. So, as hard as it may be for you, you'll probably have a better chance of getting what you want by being reasonable with her. If that doesn't work, then you might as well get angry and yell, since it may make you feel a little better—just don't expect the yelling to change anybody's mind.

Being reasonable with your parents includes a number of things. One is telling them as much as you can about what it is you want to do, so that they really understand the situation. If you simply say that you want to stay out later than usual, they may just as simply say no. If you tell them all about where you'll be and with whom and why it's important to you to stay out later (and tell them all that *before* they have a chance to say no the first time), they just might say yes. In fact, if you go on long enough giving them details about who, where, what, and why, they may get so bored hearing about it that they'll say yes just to shut you up. Anyway, it's worth a try, and it's easier than getting them to change their minds once they've already said no. Some parents really take seriously those TV spots that say, "It's ten o'clock. Do you know where your children are?" They feel guilty if they don't know. So you can relieve their anxiety and guilt by telling them in advance. Then they can talk back to the TV set.

You can sometimes use the tack with your parents of persuading them that what you want is good for you, or at least not bad for you, and that it won't make them look bad. Now I wouldn't just come out and say, "People won't think you're a bad mother if I stay late at the party." That's a little too close to the truth for some people to take. But you could say something like, "I'll just be at so-and-so's house for another hour, not wandering around the streets." That gets the point across, without making your mother feel that she has to defend her worth as a mother. With most parents, it doesn't do you any good at all to argue that you should be allowed to do something because "everybody's doing it" or because "Janie's mother lets her." The point, of course, is that you're not Janie, and your parents aren't anyone else's parents. They know perfectly well that what's reasonable for one person may not be reasonable for another. So you'll have to convince them that there are good reasons for *them* to treat *you* differently.

You may not always want to explain to your parents

what you want to do. And you have a right not to tell them about things that don't concern them. They should be willing to respect your privacy in certain areas. You have to be able to judge, in any given situation, what is important for you to keep to yourself and how much you feel comfortable telling your parents. There may be times when you have to tell them more than you really want to, and there will be other times when telling them things they don't need to know will just make your life (and theirs) more difficult. What you want to avoid is never telling them anything because you think that anything you do is none of their business. In fact, things you do sometimes do affect them. Never confiding in them about your life only leads to mistrust. They'll assume that if you can't talk about what you're doing, you must be doing something wrong.

When You Can't Agree

From time to time, nearly everyone reaches a point of complete disagreement with their parents. You are determined to do something and they are just as determined that you won't. There are two possibilities: You can either do it (whatever it is) or not. If you decide to go along with your parents' wishes, then that's all there is to it—although you may have to deal with your own feelings of resentment. If you decide that you won't or can't go along with what your parents want, then the situation becomes more complicated.

If you're going to do something that your parents don't want you to do (after being reasonable, and trying to get them to see your position, and trying to understand theirs), you can either defy them openly or else do whatever it is secretly and hope that they don't find out. The first is certainly more honest. On the other hand, it's bound to make them furious, and then you will have to deal with that. If you do what you want without telling them, you're taking the risk that they'll find out somehow. You also have to lie to them (probably), which you may or may not do well, and may not want to do. Either way, you have to try to figure out in advance what the consequences will be. Then, you have to decide if it's still worth it.

Some parents bluff a lot. If yours do, then you may know that, whatever they threaten, they won't actually do anything terrible to you. With this kind of parents, you have to be aware of the gap between what they do and what they say and not let yourself be frightened by them. Other parents really will make you stay home for three weekends just because you didn't clean up your room when you were supposed to. With parents like that, you have to try to reason with them, bargain with them, convince them that you're no longer a child, and hope that they'll eventually become more reasonable themselves. If you're not successful, there's unfortunately not much you can do about it alone. Legally, they do have control, as long as you're not being abused. However, if you feel that your parents are impossible and unreasonable, it's worth talking to someone about it—a school psychologist, guidance counselor, teacher, aunt, uncle, or older sister or brother. For some parents, it's enough to have someone they respect point out their mistakes. With others, even that doesn't work.

There *are* some bad parents. If your physical or mental health is being threatened by your parents' treatment of you, then you must get the help of someone older. Your parents' control is almost absolute, but the law protects you if your well-being is threatened. The chapter on legal rights discusses when and how to get help.

How to Get Out of Always Doing the Dishes

When it comes to household chores, the girls in a family usually get discriminated against. It's been assumed for so long by so many people that housework and child care are "women's work," that you may well find that you have to do twice as much work at home as your brother. If that's the case in your house, it's important that you try to put a stop to it. You are not physically better suited for washing dishes and wiping runny noses than your brother. You might try presenting your case to your parents first in terms of fairness. If you have to rush home from school every day to take care of your little sister while your brother hangs out with his friends, anyone should be able to see that that's an unjust situation. You can also try explaining to your parents that a more equal sharing of household chores will of course make your brother into a more responsible person.

However, keep in mind that the only thing that really concerns *you* is getting a fairer break on the chores for yourself. It's up to your parents to assign chores to your brother. Once you've expressed your thoughts about the wisdom of asking him to do his share and have gotten a fair deal for yourself, you've done all that you can do.

In some households both sons and daughters may be expected to do equal *amounts* of work, but "women's work" is assigned to girls and "men's work" to boys. It's as important for you to know how to fix appliances and do minor carpentry as it is for your brother. Volunteer for some of the chores that are "men's work" around your house—with the understanding, of course, that someone else will do the dishes while you're out mowing the lawn.

The first thing to do in bargaining with your parents about household chores is to get a clear understanding with them about just what you're responsible for. Some families make weekly or monthly lists of the household chores for which each family member is responsible. If your family is like this, then you know what's expected of you. But if you think you're being asked to do too much, or if something special comes up and you want to have an exception made, you'll still have to discuss this with your parents.

In most families, however, responsibilities are less clearly defined and depend more on the circumstances, so you'll have to keep tabs on what your parents expect you to be doing.

There are also some families where, no matter what you do, you always seem to be expected to do something different or something more. If you think all you are expected to do is wash the dishes and your mother gets angry with you because you didn't vacuum the living room, or if she always notices the one little thing you didn't do and never all the things you did, you're going to have trouble. Unless you can get the situation straightened out, you and your mother are sure to resent each other. You'll feel, and rightly so, that unfair demands are being made on you and that there's no way you can please her. She'll think you aren't living up to your responsibilities. If you have a problem like this, try to talk about it with your parents (and keep trying). If that doesn't work, you'll have to accept that your parents will never be satisfied and try not to feel guilty about that.

No matter how the chores are assigned in your family, there are certain to be special occasions when your parents need additional help or when you have something important to do and would like to be excused from your chores. You'll have to be flexible enough to be willing to help if you can when your parents need extra work done. And you'll have to explain the circumstances to them and hope they'll be reasonable and flexible in return when you need a favor.

When to Save Your Breath

There are some things that you can argue about with your parents that just aren't worth the argument. And those things may be some of the most important decisions of your life, like whether or not you're going to be a doctor or whom you're going to marry (unless you plan to get married *very* soon after the argument). But if neither of those things is going to happen immediately, you're arguing about something that doesn't depend on who "wins" the argument. It can be infuriating to have your parents make decisions (or think they're making decisions) about your life. But they can't make those long-term decisions for you unless you let them. And having a fight about something that's going to happen five years from now just doesn't make sense. Save the fights for the things that matter now.

It's important to keep in mind that your parents have moods and problems and aches and pains and things on their minds that have nothing to do with you. So if your mother snaps at you for something that you think is unimportant, it may be because she's depressed, or because she had an argument with your father, or because the phone is out of order, or just because she has a lot to do and can't figure out when she's going to get a chance to rest. When she tells you that you can't buy a skirt you want, she's not necessarily just being mean. She may be worried about an overdue electric bill or trying to figure out how to buy enough food with the money she has. It may have been a long time since she's been able to afford a new dress or something else that she wants a lot, like a vacation or just a day or two off from taking care of the house and the family.

No one is always in a good mood or a bad mood, and your parents have ups and downs just as you do. If you're having a particularly bad time with your mother or father, it can help to try to get them to talk about what's on their minds. Just talking about a problem helps most people, and if you can show someone else that you're concerned about their feelings and problems, it may help make them more sensitive to yours. Sometimes all you can do is listen; sometimes there's something that you can actually do or say to help out. Either of those may help to change your relationship with your parents on a long-term basis. Of course, talking doesn't always help, but it's certainly worth a try, especially if you and your parents usually relate to each other by fighting about everything.

Try always to keep your wits about you when you're dealing with your parents. If you can figure out where they're coming from, why they're doing what they're doing, and not accept or reject them automatically, it will make your life with them a bit easier. You shouldn't expect to learn to do that all at once, but like anything else, it gets easier with practice. If all else fails, just remember that most relationships between parents and kids improve enormously all by themselves by the time the kids are twenty-one or so. And if they haven't improved by then, you're no longer obligated to stick around.

11

Legal Rights

This chapter does not attempt to tell you everything there is to know about your individual rights as a citizen. Even if it were possible to do so, much more space than a few pages would be required to cover the subject thoroughly. Instead, I will discuss briefly some of the most common situations you could find yourself in that could lead to contact with the law. It is important to have a basic understanding of what your rights are in order to get the help you need to protect them.

Rape

There are two kinds of rape: statutory rape and forcible rape.

Statutory rape is intercourse with a woman who is below the "age of consent," whether or not she has agreed to the intercourse. The age of consent varies from state to state. Consult a current almanac to find

out what it is for your state. If you are younger than
the age of consent in your state, any boy you have
sexual intercourse with can be charged with statutory rape. The only exception is if the two of you are
married to each other.

It is unlikely that your parents would charge your
boyfriend with statutory rape if they found the two
of you having sex on the living room couch, though
they very well might give you both a lot of trouble in
other ways. They have the legal right to bring
charges against the boy, but most parents would hes-
itate to drag their daughter through a statutory rape
trial. All too often in these cases the boy's lawyer
will try to make the girl seem like a tramp, so that the
jury won't blame the boy.

Forcible rape is forced intercourse with a woman
of any age. Force, legally, includes threats of violence. In a case of forcible rape, the lawyer defending
the man often tries to gain sympathy from the jury
by claiming that the woman was behaving in a se-
ductive manner and by hinting that the poor man
couldn't help himself. Now, if you were walking
down the street with a big roll of money in your
hand and someone grabbed it from you, the robber
couldn't get away with his crime by saying that he
just couldn't resist the sight of all that money. While
it is pretty stupid to flash money around on the
street, no lawyer or jury would take the position that
the victim's stupidity was an excuse for the theft.
However, even though it's illogical, rape is the one

area of the law where the *victim* can be discriminated against in favor of the perpetrator. Many a
rapist has been freed on his own testimony that the
woman was "asking for it."

Rape is a terrifying experience for any woman.
Even the *idea* of it is terrifying, but all the same it is
a good idea to think through what you would do if it
ever happened to you. If someone is following you
or approaches you or tries to grab you, the first thing
to do is try to get away to safety. Don't run for home
if there is no one there, unless you have enough of a
lead on the man so that you're absolutely *sure* you
can get in the door and lock it behind you before he
gets there. You're better off heading for *any* place
where there are other people—a store or a neighbor's
house, for instance.

The New York City Rape Task Force recommends
that if you've been grabbed by an *unarmed* attacker
you should scream if there is any chance at all that
someone will hear you. Sometimes a rapist will just
take off as soon as the woman screams. You should
put up as much of a fight as you can—knee him in
the groin, shove your pocketbook up hard under his
chin, stamp on his feet—if there is a chance that you
can break away from him and run to safety. Some
women have been able to talk men out of raping
them, and if you're not too scared to talk, you can try
it.

If you're in a deserted place, or if you've struggled
and been overpowered, *or if you're being threatened*

with a weapon, all you can do—awful as it is—is to try to relax. Some rapists will lose interest once you stop fighting. Others will go ahead and rape you. The more you relax, the better your chances are of not being hurt by the intercourse itself. Try not to think about what's happening. Concentrate on remembering what the rapist looks like.

In order to prove rape in court, you need physical proof of intercourse, evidence that force was used, and (believe it or not) in some states you need a witness to the identity of the rapist and the fact of intercourse.

If you have been raped, the first thing you may think to do afterward may be to wash yourself and change your clothes. DON'T DO IT. You'll only be washing away evidence. The presence of semen in or near the vagina is the best possible proof that intercourse actually took place. Go straight to a hospital emergency room or a doctor. If you are too upset to get there alone, find a policeman, or anybody, and ask to be taken to a hospital. There you will be examined for signs of rape, you will be treated for any injuries you may have, and you can be given antibiotics to protect you against venereal disease and the "morning-after" pill to prevent pregnancy. You'll also have physical proof that intercourse took place and, if you were injured, that force was used.

If you have not been injured (for instance because you very reasonably gave in when threatened with a weapon), then rape will be harder to prove. It may be a difficult thing to do, but try to get a good look at the weapon so you can describe it to the police. If your attacker is later found carrying a weapon like the one you describe, you'll have a pretty good case against him.

Remember anything you can about the attacker: his face, hair, size, clothing, anything distinctive about his voice or speech. You will have to pick him out of a lineup. If you live in a state that still demands a witness to a rape, and if there wasn't one, it is sometimes possible to get the attacker charged with assault or something else if you can identify him.

When you talk to the police—as you must—after being raped, don't be surprised if they don't seem very sympathetic toward you. A lot of work has been done to improve the way authorities treat rape victims, but old habits die hard and you may be unlucky enough to be interviewed by a policeman who may ask you what you were doing out alone, or why you're wearing a short skirt, or other insulting things. Because so many police*men* have negative attitudes toward rape victims, some city police departments have set up special rape sections staffed by policewomen, who are usually easier to talk to. Many cities have women's groups who counsel rape victims and can help with legal, medical, and emotional problems. Before you need it, you should make an effort to find out if there is such a group where you live. Some hospitals give special training to their emergency room staffs in how to deal with rape victims. Aides, nurses, and doctors who have had this training will be able to help you with your feelings after the rape, as well as treat your injuries and make all the necessary reports.

Rape, although it involves sex, is not anything like healthy sexual expression. Rape is a sick act performed by men who hate women and are afraid of real sexual relationships. If you've been raped, you'll need to find someone to talk with who can help you to understand it as an isolated incident in your life. Being raped doesn't mean that you can't have a healthy sex life afterward. It doesn't mean that sex under other circumstances will be unpleasant for you.

Above all, if you've been raped, don't let *anyone* make *you* feel guilty about it. Perhaps you were unwise to have got yourself into a situation where you were raped. Or the whole thing may have been completely beyond your control. Whatever the circumstances, there is *no excuse* for a man to rape a woman. Women have the right not to be raped and, if raped, the right to be treated with the same respect victims of any other type of crime would receive. As difficult as it may be for you (and it's perfectly understandable that you may simply want to forget the whole thing), you have a responsibility to report the rape and follow it through. If you don't, the man is likely to rape again.

Juvenile Law

Until a person reaches the age of majority (the age at which you acquire the legal rights of an adult), he or she is in most respects the responsibility of adults. Parents are required by law to feed, clothe, and house you, send you to school, and take care of your other basic needs until you are old enough to provide for yourself. The age of majority is being lowered from twenty-one to eighteen in many states now that eighteen-year-olds have the right to vote. Any current almanac will tell you how old you must be in your state to gain the rights of an adult.

Until you reach the age of majority, you are considered a minor, and the law that applies to minors varies from state to state. There are only a few federal laws and Supreme Court decisions that apply to minors everywhere. Until the twentieth century there was no distinction made between juveniles and adults in criminal cases and even very young children were tried, convicted, and imprisoned (occasionally even put to death) like adult criminals. As people gradually became horrified by this system, juvenile courts and reformatories were developed to separate young offenders from adults. Most states also have special courts to deal with civil cases in which minors are involved. This separation was meant to protect young people. In general, juvenile offenders are tried in juvenile courts where the procedures are less formal than in adult courts. The judge is allowed to decide cases according to what he or she thinks is best for the defendant's welfare, and does not have to hear cases or render decisions strictly according to law. This judicial freedom was designed to allow judges to decide cases according to what they felt would most benefit the young person being tried.

Unfortunately, the system also led to abuses. In many states until very recently, young people brought into juvenile court had almost no rights and were simply at the mercy of the judge. Juveniles were not permitted to have legal representation or to call witnesses to defend themselves. This usually meant that a young person's fate was decided by whether the judge believed the defendant or the arresting officer. Guidelines on sentencing are usually vague in most juvenile courts, and it is common for the judge alone to decide what happens to the defendant. There have been cases of juveniles being sent to a reformatory until they were twenty-one years old for offenses that an adult couldn't be jailed for at all.

In recent years, some of the legal protections available to adults have been extended to minors by a series of state and federal court decisions. In 1967, in a case called *in re Gault* (Latin for "in the case of Gault"), the Supreme Court said that minors have the right to have a lawyer present at any hearing at which they are accused of a crime and face a loss of liberty. (In juvenile court it's called a hearing instead of a trial.) Juveniles also have the right to written notice of the charges against them, the right to remain silent, the right to confront their accuser, and the right to call witnesses in their own defense. A later decision called *in re Winship* makes it necessary for minors to be proved guilty *beyond a reasonable doubt*—the same standard of guilt that applies in adult courts. Before this decision it was necessary only that most of the evidence *indicated* you might be guilty. Under the *Winship* ruling, there has to be some real evidence that you actually did whatever you're accused of. You can't be convicted, for instance, just because you were seen running from the scene of a crime.

In many states, the juvenile courts still do not abide by the *Gault* or *Winship* rulings. However, since these are Supreme Court decisions, *all* juvenile courts in the United States are technically supposed to make decisions according to these guidelines. If you find yourself in juvenile court, and you feel that your rights have been violated, you should immediately get to a lawyer and discuss the situation. In large towns and cities, there are Legal Aid or state Legal Services offices or branches of the American Civil Liberties Union. They all offer free or low-cost legal help. If you are not allowed to take notes during the hearing, you should write down everything you can remember just as soon as you leave the hearing room. Among the things a lawyer will want to know are: the name and badge number (if possible) of the arresting officer, the specific charges, the names of witnesses, and as much of what was said in the hearing as you can recall. If your rights *have* been violated, there's a good chance that a higher court will reverse the ruling of the juvenile court, and you could be spared years in a reformatory.

In addition to the formal decisions about the rights of minors, the trend of recent decisions in the lower courts has been to extend the rights of juveniles and grant them more of the protections traditionally reserved for adults. However, this isn't always the case, and it is impossible to generalize for all states and all cases.

Trouble in School

The likeliest place for a minor to get into trouble is in school. School administrations in many states have, or think they have, almost absolute control over you while you are on school property. However, while school administrations have the right to make and enforce rules to maintain order, there have been certain restrictions placed on them. In general, if the penalty with which you're being threatened is serious or unreasonable, you have certain rights. Suspension for more than ten days or expulsion (or indefinite suspension, which is the same as expulsion) are considered serious penalties. If you're being threatened with such a penalty, you can demand a full hearing with a lawyer to represent you, written notice of the charges, and the right to confront your accuser and call witnesses. However, the "judge" at this hearing will probably be the school principal, who may not be totally impartial. Since in most states you are required by law to stay in school until you're sixteen or have graduated, a public school can't refuse to take you except under extreme circumstances. Thus, if the principal's decision is to expel you, there is always the chance that a court will reverse the decision. However, for that to happen, you have to be willing to go to court.

Trouble at Home

Legally, your parents have almost absolute control over you. You must do what they tell you to do unless they tell you to do something illegal. Money that you earn is legally under their control. However, if you have earned, inherited, or been given money, although you may not touch it without their permission until you are of age (or possibly even older under the terms of a will), it must be held in trust for you. Your parents can't spend it except for your benefit, and then usually only with court permission. Trusts and courts aren't usually involved, however, unless the amount of money is quite large. If you're making five dollars a week from baby-sitting, you'll have to work out on your own any conflict you may have with your parents over how it is spent.

Your parents have an obligation to support you, and they can't disown you (unless they're penniless themselves) until you are of age. In some states, however, they can rid themselves of their obligation to you by swearing in court that you are "uncontrollable" or "incorrigible" (which means that you can't be corrected). If that happens, the court can order you sent to reform school until you're twenty-one even though you've committed no crime. If ever you are faced with that, get a lawyer. There may be things you can do to protect yourself, depending on the circumstances of your case.

The only way your parents can have their rights over you taken from them is to have it proved in court that they have abused you physically, mentally, or sexually. If you feel that you're being abused by your parents, you have to get an older person—a relative or friend or lawyer—to go into court and have you removed from your parents' custody. You'll probably need a lawyer to help you get the evidence you need to prove your case.

Once you're removed from your parents' custody, the court will appoint a guardian for you for as long as you're still a minor. Your parents will still be financially responsible for your upkeep. In most states, you have some say over who your guardian is going to be. However, in some states, once you're removed from your parents' custody, you can be put in a reform school or detention home. Since many of these are worse than almost any home could be, you should check out this possibility before going into court, and try to find someone who will agree to let you live with them as long as necessary. If you are being seriously abused at home, however, it's a good idea to talk to a teacher you trust or to a guidance counselor, school psychologist, clergyman, social worker, or lawyer.

In a few states, if you are over a certain age (which varies from state to state) and you are self-supporting, you are considered an emancipated minor. This status limits your parents' rights over you and gives you certain rights of your own. In some places, even though you are supporting yourself, your parents can still go to court to force you to return home, but many courts will refuse to hear cases of this kind. However, as an emancipated minor, you still don't have all the rights of an adult, and you may have to be careful about what you do. For instance, a self-supporting woman who is under legal age can be charged as a delinquent and sent to reform school for "promiscuity" in some states. Promiscuity can mean simply that there's evidence that you've had sexual relations with one person. However, as an emancipated minor, you can rent an apartment, make certain kinds of contracts, and get medical care without your parents' knowledge or consent.

Marriage

There is one other way for a minor girl to become emancipated (at least from her parents) and that is to get married. In most states, girls can marry at eighteen without their parents' consent. You need their consent, and sometimes court approval as well, to

marry below this age. Once you are married, your
parents can no longer legally tell you what to do.
However, in some cases, your husband *can* tell you
what to do, and you may find that instead of gaining
your freedom, you've only changed masters. For instance, if you got married because your parents were
moving somewhere that you didn't want to go, and
then your husband decided to move too, you could
be legally required to go with him. Whether the passage of the Equal Rights Amendment to the Consti-
tution will have much effect on your husband's
rights over you remains to be seen. If you're under
eighteen and married, you still don't have all the
rights of an adult. In most states, you can't even sue
for divorce by yourself. You have to get an older
person to go into court as your representative (although often your lawyer will do this).

If you do manage to get married without your parents' consent when you are under legal age (either
by lying about your age or by going to a state where
the age is lower), your parents can get the marriage
annulled with no trouble at all. In some states, if
you go to another state where the age of consent is
lower and then return to your home state, your marriage won't be considered valid.

Contracts

If you sign a contract while you are a minor, that
contract cannot be enforced (with certain exceptions
discussed later). That means that if you sign a con-

tract to buy something on credit, for instance, and later you decide that you don't want it, the seller has to take back the merchandise and refund your money. Of course, if the item has been used or damaged, you won't get all your money back. But an adult has to continue to pay for an item, unless it is defective, once he has signed a contract to do so, and the seller is not required to take it back. The exception to the contract rule is that if you are over eighteen (or occasionally over sixteen) and in business for yourself, a contract that you sign in the course of your business is legally enforceable. You also can't break a marriage contract, if it was legally made, except by getting a divorce. And you can't break a contract to serve in the armed forces or a contract to obtain a driver's license. If you are contemplating signing a contract to appear as a performer or an athlete or to write a book or sell a work of art, you should consult a lawyer who specializes in that particular field.

Once you have a driver's license, you have the same liability as an adult. If you are not insured (or if you're driving without a license even in an insured car), you are personally responsible for paying any judgment against you for damages. If there is a judgment against you, your earnings for the next twenty years can be applied to pay the sum that the court decides.

Getting Busted

There are certain rights that everyone has when

arrested. These rights are absolute, and you have them no matter what the circumstances of your arrest. They apply to minors as well as to everyone else. You should know what these rights are and be able to remember them when you're under stress, which you probably will be if you're ever arrested.

The main thing to remember is that you have the right to remain silent. You have to give your name and address and the name of your parent or guardian and NOTHING ELSE. The police are supposed to tell you that you have the right to remain silent, but sometimes they don't. Whether they tell you or not, however, you shouldn't tell them anything. If they haven't advised you of your rights, you have a chance of having your case thrown out of court by the judge.

Anything you say may be used against you in a trial, which is the primary reason why you shouldn't say anything. Don't lie, don't get into conversations, don't make jokes. Sometimes the police will try to get information from you by acting friendly, or by telling you they already know what happened, or that it will go better for you in court if you level with them, or that a friend has already talked so you might as well too. Sometimes they tell you that your rights don't apply because you're too young or because you're under arrest. Sometimes they threaten you. One classic technique is to have one officer act threatening while another is friendly and protective, in the hope that you'll confide in the "nice" one. DON'T TALK.

The next thing to remember while you're sitting in the police station being quiet is that *you have a right to have a lawyer.* You should be allowed to make at least one telephone call. If you know a lawyer, call her or him directly. If not, call your parents or someone responsible and have them get a lawyer to you as soon as possible. If you can't afford to pay a lawyer, you can get one free through Legal Aid, Legal Services, or the Public Defender's office. Remember the name and badge number of the arresting officer, and tell your lawyer when he or she arrives. If the proper arresting officer doesn't show up when you're brought to court, your case can be dismissed, so it's important to remember all you can.

You should ask the arresting officer on what charge you've been arrested. If the officer refuses to answer, remember that and tell your lawyer. You have the right to know the charges against you. However, don't put up a fuss, no matter what you've been told or not told.

It's also important to remember as much as possible of what goes on at the scene of your arrest and at the police station before your lawyer arrives. You won't be allowed to write anything down, so you'll have to rely on your memory. All sorts of things that are said (and not said) and done can be important. You should tell your lawyer exactly what happened as soon as she or he arrives. Your lawyer can take notes, which are confidential, and will know what is important and what isn't to your defense.

12

Going On from Here

Books for teenagers usually sound as though they exist outside of history, as though everything that they describe has always been that way and will always be that way. *This* book is being written in 1976, eight years after the rebirth of the women's movement in this country. Since I've been a part of that movement, this book naturally reflects that. Your lives will be lived in the context of women's changing role in the society. Your life, your choices, the world you inhabit are very different from your mother's, and you are growing up at a time when the old ways of doing things are no longer adequate.

Just as this book could not have been written five years ago, some things in it will probably be out of date five years from now. No one can accurately predict how the economic, political, and social changes that are in process now will develop in the long run. These changes are going to affect all of us, women and men, in ways that are impossible to foresee. Our attitudes toward work and money, the ways in which we think about and live our family lives, the role of schools, the ways that we bring up our children will be as drastically different in ten years as they are now from ten years ago. You will have to cope with a world in which you have very few examples from the past to go by.

When you're making plans for your future, remember that almost *any* decision can be changed. There are a few people who, from early childhood, have some talent or interest that is developed into a life's work. Most of us aren't so lucky, and we try different things and change courses several times in our lives, which doesn't have to be a bad thing. You can go to school, drop out, get married, go to work, go to school some more, and you may be better off for it. Those changes should be seen by you, not as setbacks or as time lost, but as growth and progress.

A lot of us seem to have the idea that we have to make final decisions about our lives while we're in high school, or at least by the second year of college. In fact, that's not true at all. Unless you're in one of the performing arts (where early and long training is almost a necessity, although there are striking exceptions even there), you can start in science and switch to art, for example, at almost any point without having lost anything. Try to think of your education as providing choices, and keep it as wide open as you can. Learn to type, to speak a foreign language, take some math and science courses, some art, some music, some shop courses if you can get them. Give yourself the broadest possible background to work from. Then, if you do decide to change horses in midstream, you'll at least have some idea of how to handle the new horse.

You should by all means make plans and decisions and take them seriously. If you want to be a dentist, then you have to work hard in high school and college and dental school and become the best dentist you can be. At some point, when you're seventeen or thirty or forty-five or sixty, you may decide that you don't want to be a dentist anymore, that you'd be happier working in an office or being an artist. You can *always* change direction. But in the meantime, you have to do whatever you're doing as well as you possibly can.

You are going to need to be able to take care of yourself, and you can't do that very well if you go directly from your family's home to your husband's, from a situation where your parents are responsible for your welfare to a situation where your husband is. You want to break the cycle of someone else's being responsible for you and in effect owning you. Knowing that you can earn a living, make your own decisions, and take care of all the little details of your life will give you a sense of independence and confidence that you'll never lose.

If you're planning to move out of your parents' house, be as reasonable as you can with them. Explain that you're not moving out to spite them or because you don't like them. You're simply moving out in order to be on your own. They'll almost certainly come to accept the situation in time, even if they don't at first.

Whether you are going to live alone or with other people, you want to get yourself into a situation where no one is telling you what to do on your own time. When there's always someone telling you what you can and cannot do, where you can and cannot go and when and with whom, you're never going to get the chance to find out what *you* really want to do. If you're not allowed to go to a particular place, you're never going to find out if you really like going there or not—but it's always going to have the lure of the forbidden.

Had I been writing this as recently as three years ago, I'd have suggested that, once you complete your education, you move out of your parents' house, get yourself a job of some kind, and live alone for a while. You'd learn that you were capable of taking care of yourself, that you could be financially independent, that you could meet your own material needs. Then, later in your life, if you found yourself in the position of having to take care of yourself— and possibly others as well—you'd know that you were capable of doing that, from your own direct experience.

But this isn't 1973 anymore, it's 1976. And for many of you, living completely on your own isn't possible because of the changes in economic conditions over the past two years. It has simply become too expensive. But you don't have to think in conventional terms about your future. You certainly don't have to continue to live with your parents until you find a man who's willing to support you. You can think about living with a group of people as an alternative. This may be seen simply as a way to split the cost of rent or as something more. The people you live with—a group of women or a mixed group—can form a social group and a support group. You'll still be in a situation where no one can tell you what to do with your time or your money (as long as you've fulfilled your obligations to the group). Yet you'll be learning to live with other people on an equal basis, you'll have a ready source of help when you need it, and you'll be able to give help to the others. Self-reliance is not something that develops overnight. Self-reliance comes slowly with the realization that you have become strong enough and flexible enough to deal with and survive the circumstances of your life, whatever those may turn out to be. Part of the strength you need lies in the ability to ask for help from others, the ability to be open with others, to trust and depend on other people.

Many of us have been taught from the time that we were very young that someday we'd have a man to take care of us. And "taking care" meant much more than simply providing material things. We've been led to believe that the right man can fill all our social and emotional needs as well. But no one person can do that. Even if you do marry or have some other kind of long-term relationship with someone, you can't expect that person to be *everything* to you. If nothing else, that's asking entirely too much of any one human being, burdening him or her with complete responsibility for *your* happiness. Having a group of people that you depend on, having close friendships with several people, whether or not you live with them, means that if one person leaves or one relationship falls apart, you aren't left alone.

Just as you don't have to put all your emotional energies into one person, you don't have to put all your creative energies into any one part of your life. You can live with people, get married, continue your education (in school or on your own), have a job, have children. You can do any combination of those things that suits you, and no one part of your life has to become so important that it leaves no room for the rest.

The world is changing and you have the choice of taking an active part in that change or of just letting it happen to you. If you're not happy with the world as it is, if you're not content about the direction that things seem to be going, then you have a responsibility to take part in changing things to the way you want them to be. None of us can do that alone, but taking an active part in history may be the greatest satisfaction that any of us can have in a difficult time.

For most people, the teenage years are a period of

marking time, a time of waiting to grow up, waiting for life to begin. It's a time when many of us feel acted upon by demands and forces that we have no control over. But these years don't have to be a waste of time. These can be the years when you start to learn about yourself and the world around you in a conscious and active way. You can look at the future you want and start to work toward it, remembering that the future and the present are continuous. This *is* your life, so you might as well stop waiting for it to start.

Additional and Recommended Reading

Babcox, Deborah, and Belkin, Madeline. *Liberation Now.* New York: Dell Publishing Co., 1971.

The Boston Women's Health Book Collective. *Our Bodies, Ourselves.* 2nd ed., rev. New York: Simon & Schuster, 1976.

Brownmiller, Susan. *Against Our Will.* New York: Simon & Schuster, 1975.

Frankfort, Ellen. *Vaginal Politics.* New York: Quadrangle Books, 1972.

Hansen, Soren, and Jensen, Jesper. *Little Red School Book.* New York: Pocket Books, 1971.

Morgan, Robin, ed. *Sisterhood Is Powerful: An Anthology of Writings from the Women's Liberation Movement.* New York: Random House, 1970.

Paulsen, Kathryn, and Kuhn, Ryan A., comp. and ed. *Woman's Almanac.* Philadelphia: J. B. Lippincott Co., 1976.

Strouse, Jean. *Up Against the Law: The Legal Rights of People Under 21.* New York: New American Library, 1970.

Weideger, Paula. *Menstruation & Menopause: The Physiology and the Psychology, the Myth and the Reality.* New York: Alfred A. Knopf, 1976.

The following pamphlets by the Health Organizing Collective and HealthRight may be obtained by writing to: HealthRight, Women's Health Forum, 175 Fifth Avenue, New York, N.Y. 10010.

The Gynecological Check-Up
Health Story (your personal medical record)
Infections of the Vagina
Notes on Vaginal Infections (supplement to above)

Index

ANDREA BOROFF EAGAN was born in New York City, attended Bennington College, and graduated from Columbia University in 1969. She has been active in various aspects of the women's movement, has taught "Know Your Body" courses to numerous women's groups, and currently is at work on a book that focuses on the experience of the mother in the first months after the birth of a baby. She lives with her husband and young daughter in Brooklyn, New York. *Why Am I So Miserable If These Are the Best Years of My Life?* is her first book.

ELLEN FRANKFORT is the author of *Vaginal Politics*.